HEART AND VECTOR

Physical basis of electrocardiography

HEART AND VECTOR

Physical Basis of
Electrocardiography

H. C. BURGER

editor:

H. W. JULIUS Jr.

PHILIPS TECHNICAL LIBRARY

GORDON AND BREACH, SCIENCE PUBLISHERS INC.

This book contains xii + 142 pages, 78 illustrations

Library of Congress Catalog Card Number 68-59191

 PHILIPS

Trademarks of N.V. Philips' Gloeilampenfabrieken

Distributors for the U.S.A. and Canada:
GORDON AND BREACH, Science Publishers Inc.
150 Fifth Avenue, New York, N.Y. 10011

Printed in the Netherlands

FOREWORD

With feelings of gratitude I have accepted the request of the publishers and of the Editor of this book, to write a short introduction. "Heart and Vector", based on the fundamental research of many scientists, both in the field of medical physics and of clinical medicine, gives a description of physical aspects of electrical phenomena of cardiac activity. It especially deals with the electrical activity as it can be observed at the surface of the living human body.

It is not up to me to mention here the names of those scientists with whom my late brother Herman C. Burger, professor of Medical Physics at the State University of Utrecht was connected with close mutual ties of scientific appreciation and cordial friendship. I simply want to state that this international cooperation in science was a definite part of his personality and that, particularly, this has enlightened his last years of scientific activity which by other reasons were so bitter for him. He often expressed to me his feelings of deep thankfulness towards all those scientists for their cooperative, open-minded and critical attitude.

Special feelings of appreciation are also conveyed to those, who have made it possible to publish this book, containing a comprehensive survey of the last course of academic lectures of medical physics at the University of Utrecht, which my brother served for approximately half a century. I feel obliged to mention here the name of one of his last pupils, H. W. Julius, who edited these lectures and prepared them for publication. I know that this work was highly appreciated by my brother.

In the preface of this book Julius presents some brief historical remarks concerning the work of H. C. Burger in the field of electrical phenomena of the activity of the heart. Here I will only add one aspect, which, I think, should be mentioned. As a worker in the field of preventive medicine and occupational health, the early detection and diagnosis and treatment of coronary heart disease aroused my special attention. It was this basic atittude that determined the special interest of my brother for physical problems of the heart's activity in general and of vectorcardiography in a more specific sense. We were both convinced that vectorcardiography, even after having got a sound physical basis, did not attract the attention, which it deserves in clinical and preventive medicine not only as a method for research and diagnosis, but also for its educational or learning value. Recent research has shown the significance of the exact knowledge of those electrical phenomena studied at the surface of the body as a basis for a better understanding and new developments in electrocardiography as a whole, including both "classic" electrocardiography and vectorcardiography. This book, therefore, deserves the interest of a large group of scientific workers: clinicians, physiologists and medical physicists.

It appears to be appropriate to point out in this introduction some of the fundamental thoughts of H. C. Burger's work in the field of medical physics. He was of the opinion that the systematic application of the physical methods of thinking, experimentation and measurement not only are of great importance, but should be considered as a fundamental condition, as a must, for an optimal development of medical science. In comparison with technical sciences, medical science, missing as one of its solid pillars full development of medical physical knowledge, should necessarily be considered as a kind of underdevelopped territory in this respect and this would not at all be to the benefit of mankind.

Possibly there will come a time when lifeless nature, being the original object of the physical science, might have to be considered as a "special case" of living nature. Although it may be so that the human spirit will never succeed to disentangle the fundamental processes of life, nevertheless man should keep trying to do so, exploring again and again new parts of the terra incognita of life. The more natural sciences will proceed on this way, the more medicine will be *science* and shift its quality of an *art* to another level of thinking. The higher the level of scientific knowledge will be, the more there will remain a need and a possibility for a successful humanitarian approach to the sufferings of mankind.

At the end of this introduction votes of thank have to be conveyed towards the Centrex Publishing Company for its willingness to publish this book.

This company recently (1965) published the book: Vectorcardiography. The author, J. B. Boutkan, physician, presents, after a brief physical introduction, the *clinical* aspects of the method.

"Heart and Vector" now describes the *physical* aspects of the method in a fundamental and detailed way. Together, these two books give a full picture of one of the important new developments in cardiology.

G. C. E. Burger

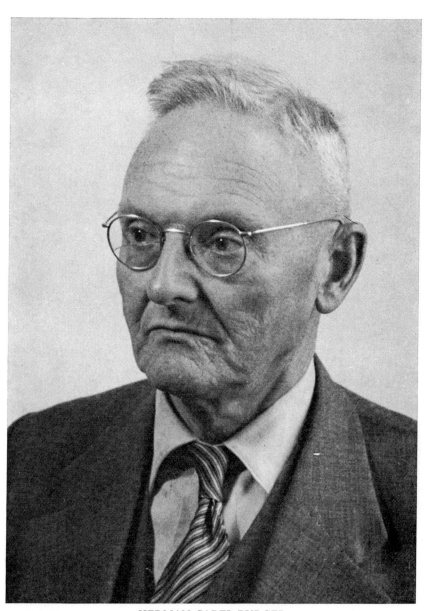

HERMAN CAREL BURGER

PREFACE

In 1964, at the end of the academic year, professor H. C. Burger retired under the superannuation-limit as professor of medical-physics of the State University of Utrecht, Holland. The course of lectures he gave during the last year of his tenure of office has been recorded in this book. It is not a coincidence that Burger chose vectorcardiography as the last topic to deal with before his retirement. Since he won himself an excellent reputation in this field — and beyond it! — it may be interesting to mention some historical facts.

When Burger, in 1911, intended to go to the university, three subjects of study were considered: physics, medicine and biology, all three belonging to his sfere of interest. At last his love for physics prevailed, in spite of the fact that, according to the law of those days, he was obliged to qualify in classics, before he would be allowed to take exams in that subject. Although with aversion, he overcame this barrier in a very short time.

In 1918 Burger finished his studies with honors on a thesis concerning the solving and growing of crystals ("Oplossen en groeien van kristallen"), under supervision of his promotor L. S. Ornstein, professor of theoretical physics of the State University of Utrecht. The choice of the subject, which was in between theoretical and experimental physics and which touched physical chemistry, may be seen as the first indication of Burger's interest in working in comprehensive but fascinating confines.

Apart from a period of $2\frac{1}{2}$ years — in which he was active in the physical laboratory of Philips Ltd. in Eindhoven, Holland — Burger was on the staff of the physical laboratory of the Utrecht State University for his entire scientific carrier of half a century, in spite of several invitations from other universities.

His interest in medical science was kept alive, on the one hand by the fact that, as a lecturer, it was his task to give lectures in physics for medical students, prospective biologists etc., on the other hand by the intensivating scientific contact he had with his brother, G. C. E. Burger, who did study medicine. These very contacts have prompted him in the direction of the confines of both sciences. This resulted, among other things, in the publication of a book about "Medical Physics" (1949), which was edited by both the Burger brothers.

Also his interest in vectorcardiography is a result of the scientific contact with his brother. It seems to be worthwhile to say somewhat more about this.

Already some years before World War II, Philips — of the health center of which G. C. E. Burger was in charge — received a request to occupy themselves with the realisation of a patent of which the patentees were a german physicist and a physician and which was granted on a new method of electrocardiography: by means of potential measurements on the body surface, they tried to gather some knowledge concerning the so-called "heart-vector" — a conception that was introduced earlier by Einthoven, under the name "manifest value" — to make the data subservient to clinical diagnosis. Naturally G. C. E. Burger, the medical man, was concerned in the investigation. While studying this subject, which was new for Philips, he set eyes on many publications. Some of these induced him to propound the following problem to his brother, the physicist:

"Look at this equilateral triangle with the human figure in it, quote from cardiological literature (see Fig. 9, page 18). The angular point of the triangle represent the three electrodes according to Einthoven on right arm, left arm and left foot. The arrow drawn inside the heart, the heartvector, represents an instantaneous view of the electrical heart action. Now the author of the article, in which all this is explained, shows how one can determine the potential differences for this moment, by means of this image, by constructing the projections of the heartvector on the sides of the triangle. In a reversed order it is possible, in practice, to decide on the heartvector from the measured differences of potential between the successive limb electrodes.

How inviting this may be, there must be something wrong, for, conceived in this way, magnitude and direction of the heartvector would be dependent on the shape of the triangle and hence of the length of the arms!"

Burger, the physicist, not only agreed with the criticism of his brother, but also let himself easily be persuaded to examine in which concrete form this conception could be moulded without coming into conflict with physics. In this way, as it was to appear, a long series of experiments began for Burger in the field of vectorcardiography, which were to lead not only to a firm physical foundation of this special method, but also to a better comprehension of the more general electrocardiography.

On the basis of these fundamental medical-physical investigations, in the physical laboratories of the Utrecht State University as well as of Philips Ltd., vectorcardiographs were built to be tested in clinical practice.

Burger's investigations did not confine themselves to this field only, he also paid attention to many other medical problems in which physics come into action. In 1951 he was appointed professor, so that the foundation of a self-supporting department of medical-physics could be realised. As the head of this department he has done pioneering work and made himself one of the pillars of today's medical physics.

Burger was particularly zealous for a firm cooperation between physician and physicist. Although his fabulous acuteness, complete integrity and his frankness did not always appear to be the right matrix for combined deliberation — a consequence of the fact that he lacked the qualities of a subtle tactician — he convinced many workers of the desirability, sometimes the necessity, to meet in the confines of the sciences. It is with him that medicine now develops as a science rather than as an art. For, he was in the position to exercise influence on many generations of medical men in the sense of introducement of a more exact approach in clinical circles. Just as well the generations of medical-physicists will regard him as a shining example, because his thoughts were of the most pure kind. I feel grateful that I was in the position of having been one of his latest disciples.

As mentioned above, Burger devoted his last course of lectures to giving a general view of physical aspects in electrocardiography (at which he did not fail to emphasize vectorcardiography). He asked me to put the whole thing on paper. There were two reasons for it:

The first had its origin in the desire of some american prominents in the field of vectorcardiography and Burger, to compile, in mutual cooperation, a book which should give a general survey of all that is important in the field. The fact that it appeared to be impossible to realize this project within a reasonable period of time, has given rise to the suggestion to publish Burger's lectures separately.

Second: In 1965 "Centrex Publishing Company" published the book "Vectorcardiography" by J. Boutkan, M. D. This book, which is written from a pure clinical point of view, naturally gives the head-lines of the physical background. Nevertheless, it seemed to be profitable to elucidate the physics of electrocardiography from the physicist's point of view, in a parallel publication. It was obvious for this to make use of H. C. Burger's wide information and experience.

In that capacity this book — in which problems concerning choice of systems and physical foundation of some systems (among which is the B(urger) system, used by J. Boutkan) are described — is to be considered.

When I had finished the text, Dr H. C. Burger and I discussed the whole manuscript, a work that I shall remember as one of the most pleasant I have ever done. Now the result is presented to the reader in a form to which Burger has given his approval. I mention with deep regret that his death prevented him from being a witness of the publication of this book.

I thank professor M. T. Jansen for his contribution regarding histological and anatomical aspects of the subject (Chapters 3 and 15) and also G. van Herpen, M.D., who took the responsibility for the last chapter.

Utrecht 1967   H. W. Julius Jr.

CONTENTS

CHAPTER 1

INTRODUCTION

The discovery, many years ago, of the electrical phenomena associated with the heartbeat led to the development of electrocardiography and the electrocardiogram (ECG). By this electrophysiological method the clinician can assess heart function and study certain pathological aberrations.

The basic principle is the measurement of differences of potential between various points on the surface of the body as a function of time during the cardiac cycle; the ECG is a diagrammatic representation of these potential differences.

A variation on this principle, the vectorcardiography and the vectorcardiogram (VCG), will here be considered in more detail. However, one has to bear in mind that vectorcardiography and electrocardiography cannot be clearly separated from one another as they are so closely related.

A problem may be approached from two points of view: the analytic and the synthetic. Using the analytic method we shall first investigate the various electrical phenomena on the body surface associated with the heart beat. At the end we shall penetrate into the heart as source of electricity.

The history of electrocardiography is of help when we study the development of this technique as well as when we attempt to understand the misconceptions which have arisen in connection with the subject. These misconceptions have in part arisen because of the difficulty of combining less precise biological methods with more exact physical concepts.

Before we discuss the fundamental physical problems relating to electrocardiography and vectorcardiography we shall consider the instrumentation n the next chapter.

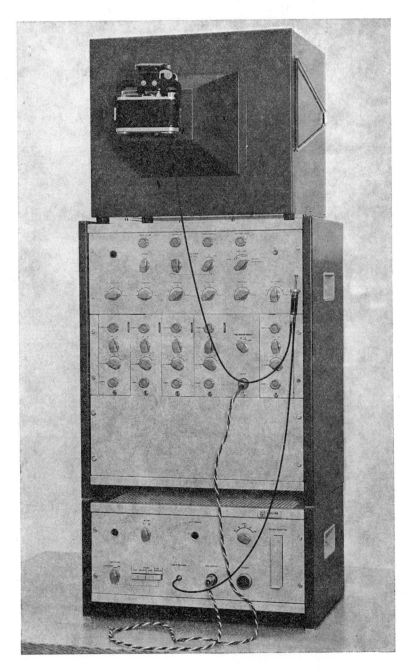

Philips vector-cardiograph built up with the components for the systems Burger-Wilson, Frank and Mac Fee. The system units are interchangeable by means of plug-in printed circuits. An empty print is supplied with the apparatus as to enable user to incorporate other systems in the vector-cardiograph.

CHAPTER 2

USE OF INSTRUMENTS
IN ELECTROCARDIOGRAPHY

2.1. General

As a result of electrical activity taking place in the heart, an electrical phenomenon takes place on the surface of the body. This phenomenon varies in place and time with the cardiac cycle. In electrocardiography some measurement of these electrical phenomena must be made.

Whether current or voltage should be measured was a subject of discussion for many years. It has now been decided that voltage is the *only* feature to measure, for to measure current it is necessary to interrupt the circuit for the introduction of an ammeter and this is *not* possible with a medium such as the human body.

The electrocardiogram is therefore based on the measurement of voltages, hence of potential *differences*. A certain amount of controversy has occured with reference to this measurement too: some workers considered that knowledge of the actual potential at any one point was important, whereas today it is widely realised that this information, even if we could get it, has no meaning. This can be demonstrated by the fact that the potential difference between any couple of points (and hence the heart function) is not affected by exposing the body to a million volts with reference to earth! Notwithstanding that, some workers are still influenced by this controversy, to the extend that they use methods whereby potential differences are measured between all points of interest and one meticulously selected reference point at which a constant or even a zero potential is valued (see page 13).

Before we go more deeply into the details of the method and the theoretical background, we shall discuss the instruments in electrocardiography.

2.2. Properties of the electrocardiographic apparatus

The electrocardiograph is essentially a voltmeter which must fulfill certain requirements to be discussed below.

2.2.1 SENSITIVITY

The voltages which the instrument must measure are not much greater than 1 millivolt. The sensitivity of the voltmeter, defined as the deflection in mm of the indicator per unit of voltage in millivolts, must be sufficient to be satisfactory. So that comparison between ECG's obtained with different instruments is possible a uniform deflection must be agreed on. The scale used is 1 millivolt equivalent to 10 mm (see footnote page 17). It seems that this scale is in fact too small and that some detail is lost.

2.2.2 HIGH INPUT IMPEDANCE

Because this requirement is essential in all voltmeters, it must be basic in the electrocardiograph too. If the input impedance is too small, a significant current can go astray, which at the measuring point yields a voltage drop dependent upon the changing resistance of the skin, the latter being rather high (of the order of 10^5 $\Omega \cdot cm^2$). Various methods have been tried to reduce the skin resistivity: pastes readily absorbed by the skin, abrasion of the skin etc. Modern electronics, however, permit such high input impedance ($\pm$ 10 MΩ) that it is found to be sufficient to saturate the electrodes (furnished with small foam rubber pads) with NaCl solution which penetrates the outer layer of the skin and thus effects an electrolytic contact.

In addition to the normal ohmic skin resistance, another phenomenon makes a high input impedance necessary, and that is electrolytic polarization. This causes a counteracting electromotive force on the surface of the electrodes which in good approximation is proportional to the total amount of electricity flowing through ($\int i dt$).

2.2.3 SHORT INDICATING TIME

Although a complete heart cycle takes about one second, the various changes in this period occur so rapidly that the requirement for quick action in the instrument is high. This property is needed not only by the mechanical part of the recording apparatus but also for the electronic part of it (amplifiers), so that fast voltage changes can be transmitted without distortion. One can argue about the frequencies at which undistorted reproduction is required. Opinions on this are divergent, but it is industry that "helps" us out of the impasse here and in practice seldom sets the limit above 500 to 1000 cycles per second. (Can anybody derive any valuable information above these frequencies . . . ?)

The frequency and jump characteristics offer complete information on the performance of the apparatus in this respect.

It is not sufficient, of course, that the electrocardiograph itself should work rapidly; it is also necessary for the speed of movement of film or paper strip to be such that quick changes can be recorded. A uniform and generally satisfactory speed, necessary for purposes of comparison and resolving power, is fixed at 25 mm/sec (see footnote page 17). In special circumstances this rate may be increased by a factor ot 2, 4 or even 10.

The sharpness and thickness of the pen or ink jet tracing must also be considered. The thinner the line, the more information in proportion to the area of the paper.

2.2.4 EXTERNAL CONDITIONS CAUSING ARTEFACTS

These, of course, must always be guarded against when using instruments of physical measurement. We shall not discuss this subject in detail except in so far as the electrocardiograph is affected.

a. Electrical disturbances:

In principle these can be overcome in large measure today by the balanced input of the electronic part of the apparatus. Sometimes practice proves however that, notwithstanding this supply, disturbances are not always satisfactory depressed. An effective solution of the problem, but which in the clinic is impractical, is to surround the patient, electrodes, leads and pre-amplifier with a Faraday cage.

b. Magnetic disturbances:

Caused for examle by rotating motors. Here also, as under section (a), screening should be constructed of a material with high magnetic permeability, though the high cost makes this practically impossible. Besides, the stress effect of gadgeting on the patient will probably produce a greater disturbance than we are attempting to eliminate! (see section (d)). The measures that can be taken are: remain as far as possible from the source, avoid use of straps, or, in application of "counter-straps", try for a compensation. Sometimes only one measure helps: cut off the source.

c. Building vibrations:

These may be transmitted to the recorder via the tubes of the electronic apparatus.

d. Muscular movement:

Not only heart activity gives rise to potential differences on the body surface, the activity of all muscles is associated with electrical phenomena. To avoid the effect of other muscles on the electrocardiogram it is therefore necessary to see that the patient is as relaxed as possible. He should be allowed to lie down and care must be taken to put him at his ease. The room temperature must be comfortable so that shivering (involuntary muscular contraction) does not occur. It is difficult to presuade small children to keep still and this makes recording from them particularly difficult.

e. Poor contacts:

Shifting or loosening of the electrodes, or drying of the electrolyte, can completely ruin a tracing.

Modern techniques have gone so far towards solving all the above problems that electrocardiography can be more and more easily undertaken during the course of routine work.

Less essential but desirable properties which should also be assessed may be considered together and include sturdy construction, ease of operation, reliability, pleasing appearance, lightness and moderate price.

2.3 Historical development of the electrocardiograph

We shall now briefly consider the instruments which have been used over the years, and see how they have developed to reach the present satisfactory state.

The old multiplier (forerunner of the galvanometer) can be ignored for it was merely able to indicate qualitatively the existence of an electrical effect during the cardiac cycle.

The first usable instrument was

2.3.1 THE CAPILLARY ELECTROMETER

This instrument was invented by Lippmann in 1873, in Paris. In its simplest form it consists of a thin U-tube filled with mercury and sulphuric acid and provided with two electrodes (Fig. 1). Even a small potential difference across the two electrodes causes polarisation at the junction of the two liquids; the resultant change in surface tension causes a movement of the mercury meniscus. The direction of this movement depends on the polarity of the

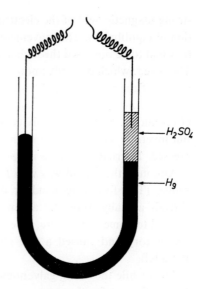

Fig. 1. Lippmann's capillary electrometer

H_2SO_4

Hg

applied voltage and the deflection is approximately proportional to it. The internal resistance could be raised to high values. Recording was accomplished by means of a photographic plate.

The performance of this instrument (which meanwhile has been relegated to the museum) was far from ideal because of the great inertia and internal friction of the mercury column and we would not have mentioned it had it not been the starting point for a revolutionary development.

It remained for Einthoven — a physician! — to study the physical properties of the capillary electrometer by deriving and solving the differential equation relating to the system. He analyzed the recorded tracings mathematically and calculated the "true" ECG (later measurements confirmed his results). Dissatisfied with this cumbersome procedure and in search of a more elegant technique, he constructed

2.3.2 THE STRING GALVANOMETER

The essential feature of this instrument is a silvered or gold-plated quartz thread (the "string"), 2 to 5 μm in diameter, stretched vertically between the poles of an electromagnet.

The action of this apparatus is based on the Lorentz effect. If the voltage to be measured is connected to the two outer ends of the thread, an electric current then flows and produces a magnetic field which, interacting with the strong magnetic field of the electromagnet, deflects the thread from its position of equilibrium. The movements of the quartz thread were so slight that they had to be observed through a microscope or photographically recorded. The speed, which depends upon the natural frequency of the moving system (hence of the thickness and tension of the string) and upon damping (hence upon the magnetic field) is substantially better than that of the capillary electrometer. Also the sensitivity (likewise determined by the string tension, but inversely so and by the strength of the magnetic field) can be much increased. Internal resistance is approximately 10^4 Ω.

Although the thread was very fine, its thickness still limited its frequency range. (The following incident demonstrates how very fine Einthoven's threads actually were. All attempts to produce still more delicate strings seemed to come to a failure. One day a sunbeam accidentally penetrated the Laboratory and caused a fine glitter: the air was full of floating quartz threads!).

Meanwhile the string galvanometer has gone its way to the museum and has made way for the

2.3.3 ELECTRONIC APPARATUS

The application of electronic devices to electrocardiography constitutes a big advance. It makes it possible to meet simultaneously practically all the requirements mentioned above. First must be noted the greater input impedance (ca. 10^7 Ω), which makes the various disagreeable methods of reducing skin resistance unnecessary (see page 4). Sensitivity can now be selected at will, as a consequence of the initial unlimited possibility of amplification.

The instruments described above were themselves the indicators. Electronics, in addition to the amplifier (which formerly was used in combination with the string galvanometer) have furnished still another indicator — which by itself has a small sensitivity — namely the electron beam oscilloscope. The low value of the quotient m/e for an electron [1]) makes this apparatus so fast that the indicating time of the voltmeter as a whole is determined by the properties of the preconnected amplifier.

There are certain other favourable characteristics which are worth noting,

---

[1]) The setting time of an oscilloscope is determined by the time required for an electron to pass between the deflecting plates. The speed of travel of an electron, determined by $\frac{1}{2}mv^2 = eV$, is high, because m/e is very small.

especially when the apparatus is to be used by medical personnel rather than electronic engineers. These are: simplicity of operation, reliability (no danger that the thread will be broken if too high a stress is developed!) and low bulk (especially since the advent of the transistor).

2.4 Recording technique

This is sufficiently important a facet of the development of instruments to merit separate discussion.

Both the movement of the mercury column of the capillary electrometer and that of the thread in Einthoven's apparatus were recorded on photographic plates. The oscilloscope also makes use of this method, though optical instrumentation can be simpler. The obsolete plate is replaced today by a roll of sensitized paper.

The use of photography as a method of recording has still certain drawbacks worthy of note. First, there is the delay necessitated by the finishing process, which is a nuisance when both patient and physician are impatient to see immediate results. This delay is also a nuisance to the experimental physicist who may be unable to determine directly if a specific setting of his apparatus is accurate or not; in other words, he cannot control his machine.

The so-called direct recorders were thus clearly desirable. We shall now discuss some of these.

2.4.1 THE PEN RECORDER

The pen recorder consists of a pen with an ink reservoir at the end of a rather long arm. The rather large mass of this system means that much energy is needed to produce a certain deflection in a short time. Modern amplifiers can adequately meet this requirement, but high frequencies constitute a great problem. The natural frequency of the system can be made as high as desired, of course, but the problems arising for example from the flexibility of the arm are not solved in this way. In practice the frequency range is set at about 100 cycles per second.

2.4.2 THE HOT WIRE RECORDER

An electrically heated wire is supported on a rotating drum (Fig. 2). Over the drum there passes a strip of black paper, covered with a thin white layer of a

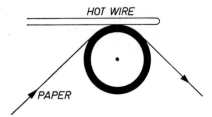

Fig. 2. The hot-wire recorder

substance with a suitably low melting point. The small contact area between wire and paper makes it possible to trace a fine and most contrasting line. A special advantage of this recorder is that the deflection is recorded parallel to the drum shaft while the pen describes an arc (see 2.4.1). For the same reasons as above, the maximum frequency here is low and does not exceed 250 cycles per second.

2.4.3 THE LIQUID JET

Ink is projected through a thin bent nozzle as a very fine jet. Because of the slight mass of the nozzle, the natural frequency can be raised to about 800 cycles per second.

An example of such a device is the "Mingograph". If the model is a multi-channel recorder, a difficulty can arise: the most minute particle of dust in the mouth of the pipe can deflect the liquid jet by a certain angle. If this deflection is in exactly the same direction as the running direction of the paper, or if it is opposed thereto, an apparent difference in time between the channels can be introduced.

2.4.4 FAST PHOTOGRAPHIC METHOD

Recently much attention has been given to the ultrafast developing of films. It is now possible to see the positive print within one minute or less of recording (Polaroid system). A further "development" in this field can be expected. UV sensitive recording paper is now available which is processed in daylight.

CHAPTER 3

THE PLACING OF THE ELECTRODES AND THE ECG

To record potential differences as a function of time (a so-called lead), two electrodes are placed anywhere on the body surface. Theoretically there are ∞^2 possible positions [1]) for these pairs of electrodes. Einthoven, the pioneer of electrocardiography, introduced uniformity into this field by regularly placing the electrodes on the right arm (R), left arm (L) and left leg (F). More precise positioning is not necessary because the electric current penetrates so little into the extremities that they can be regarded as equipotential volumes. These electrode positions constituting leads I, II and III are still used today (see Fig. 3).

3.1 Einthoven's law of summation

For the leads of any three electrodes and hence also for the limb leads Einthoven's law of summation is valid:

$$I + II + III = (V_L - V_R) + (V_R - V_F) + (V_F - V_L) = 0 \,[2]) \qquad (3.1)$$

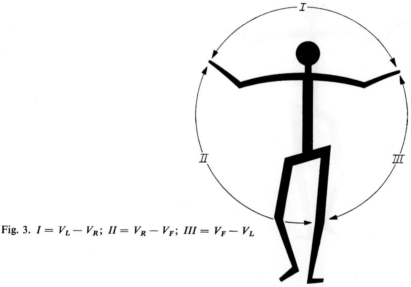

Fig. 3. $I = V_L - V_R$; $II = V_R - V_F$; $III = V_F - V_L$

---

[1]) It might be supposed that this number would be ∞^4, i.e. ∞^2 possible positions for each electrode, but clearly since we are measuring *differences* of potential the true number is ∞^2. (See also Einthoven's law of summation on this page.)

[2]) In medical literature it is customary to indicate lead II by $V_F - V_R$. Then with $II^* = -II$, Einthoven's law reads: $I + III = II^*$.

In the introduction it was noted that the answer has been sought to the question — which in the past was frequently asked in medical circles — "What about the potentials of each extremity separately?" The fact that the question, which could be solved up to a certain point, was raised, is not in itself incomprehensible, but the uncertain physical grounds on which work has previously based sounds that way. We know now that the question is meaningless, but many years passed, alas, before the physicist, in the beginning travelling slowly and hesitantly over unaccustomed terrain, was able to connect the wrong routes with the right path.

3.2 The Central Terminal

The desire to be able to measure "a potential" led meanwhile to the introduction of the so-called Central Terminal (CT) (Wilson): if the electrodes of the three extremities are connected via three equal resistances (r) (which must be large when compared with skin resistance but negligible in comparison with the input impedance of the measuring instrument) with each other (see Fig. 4) then a point, the Central Terminal, is obtained, which can be used as a reference point in the measurement of voltages on the body surface.

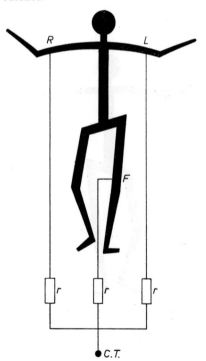

Fig. 4. The Central Terminal

In the past it was customary either to take the potential of the CT to be zero, or to assume a constant potential throughout the cardiac cycle. Both approaches were misguided. It can be said that V_{CT} at any time is the average of V_R, V_L and V_F (with reference to any point):

$$V_{CT} = \frac{V_R + V_L + V_F}{3} \tag{3.2}$$

That this is true can be seen by assuming that the input impedance of the apparatus is so great that no current passes from the CT to the apparatus. In that case, according to Kirchhoff's first law, the equation that holds is:

$$\frac{(V_R - C_{CT})}{r} + \frac{(V_L - V_{CT})}{r} + \frac{(V_F - V_{CT})}{r} = 0 \tag{3.3}$$

from which (3.2) follows immediately.

The voltage at any point on the body surface (or even in the body) can of course be measured with reference to the Central Terminal. It is for instance easy to see that

$$V_R - V_{CT} = \frac{2}{3} \frac{(V_R - V_L) + (V_R - V_F)}{2} = \frac{2}{3} \left(V_R - \frac{V_L + V_F}{2} \right) \tag{3.4}$$

Although this method is accurate it is cumbersome and no more information is obtained than when any other point on the body is chosen as reference. More can be learned if more electrodes are applied in addition to the three limb electrodes. The usual way in which these electrodes are placed in clinical practice is shown in Fig. 5.

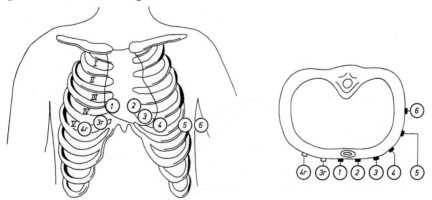

Fig. 5. Normal positioning of the electrodes

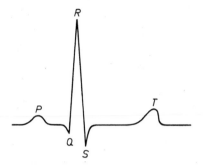

Fig. 6. Basic form of the ECG

The basic form of an electrocardiogram is outlined in Fig. 6. The use of the letters P, Q, R, S and T to designate waves is internationally accepted and was originated by Einthoven. In order to understand the significance of the electrocardiogram in terms of cardiac function we shall briefly review the anatomy.

3.3 The ECG. Anatomy of the heart

The heart is not heart shaped (Fig. 7). It is made up of right and left sections which are not identical, the left having thicker walls than the right. The right and left sections are each divisible into two parts, an atrium and a ventricle. The left and right atria and ventricles are separated from one another by the atrial septum and the ventricular septum respectively. Blood flows into the right atrium from the venae cavae, having previously passed

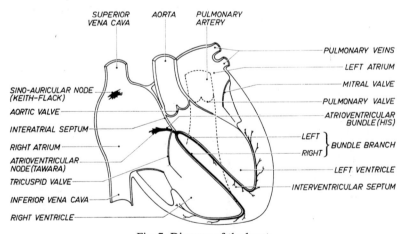

Fig. 7. Diagram of the heart

through the systemic circulation. This venous blood flows into the atrium when the ventricle is in diastole and the muscle of its wall is relaxed.

Atrial contraction helps to direct the stream of blood from the atria towards the ventricles, but one cannot speak of a true pump-mechanism since no valves are present that could prevent back flow of blood to the veins.

When ventricular systole begins the tricuspid valve is pushed closed. The connection of the cusps of the valve to the ventricular walls by tendinous cords (the chordae tendineae) prevents these cusps being inverted by the pressure of the blood during systole. These cords are attached to the tops of conical muscles jutting out into the ventricular cavity. By contracting synchronously with the other ventricular musculature they compensate for the decrease in distance from the ventricular wall to the plane of the valves. When the blood pressure in the ventricle exceeds that in the pulmonary artery the pulmonary valve, which consists of three semilunar segments or cusps, is pushed open and blood leaves the ventricle to flow into the pulmonary artery. The blood then flows to the lungs and returns to the left atrium via the pulmonary veins. From the left atrium the blood flows through the bicuspid (mitral) valve into the left ventricle and thence through the aortic valve into the aorta. Since the left ventricular contractions have to push the blood through the systemic arteries against much higher resistance than that met by the right ventricle which has only to push the blood through the pulmonary arteries the left ventricular wall is much thicker than the right (1.5 cm as against 0.5 cm).

The ventricles, by far the larger part of the heart, resemble an inverted pear in shape when both are viewed together. At the blunt end of this pear is a circular plate of connective tissue (the annulus fibrosus) where the openings of the tricuspid, bicuspid, aortic and pulmonary valves are to be found clustered together.

The chambers of the heart are lined on the inside by the smooth endocardium and on the outside by the equally smooth epicardium. The epicardium is separated by a thin film of fluid from the smooth pericardium. This construction offers a large degree of freedom of movement to the ventricles.

The blood supply to the myocardium comes from the coronary arteries which leave the aorta near its point of origin and pass just deep to the epicardium to form branches into the depth of the muscular tissue.

Contraction of the myocardium is not, as is the case of all other muscles, caused by an impulse from the nervous system. The heart (Fig. 7) has its own pacemaker, the sinu-atrial node (Keith-Flack) which is a part of the myocardium with a characteristic undifferentiated structure. A stimulus from this pacemaker can spread over the muscular wall of the atrium in a very short time and cause its contraction. Excitation of the atrium stimulates the atrio-ventricular node (Tawara), from which, via the atrio-ventricular bundle of His-Tawara (which penetrates the non-conducting connective tissue of the annulus fibrosus between the atria and the ventricles) the impulse is further transmitted to the ventricles. In the ventricles this transmitting system bifurcates into the two so-called bundle branches along the endocardial sides of the septum and from these a finer branching system of fibres (the Purkinje system) conducts the stimulus to the myocardium. The muscle tissue itself transmits the stimulus further from cell to cell.

Electrical activity in the heart occurs in the following manner. The excited part of the myocardium is adjacent to that part in which activity is yet to occur. The potentials of these two parts are different, that of the excited part being lower than that of the other. Thus an electric field is established, varying in time and place within the cardiac cycle. (The above will be discussed in detail in Chapter 15.)

The ECG can now be interpreted as follows:

P wave: represents atrial contraction (the electrical activity is a spread of excitation or depolarisation through the atrium).

PQ interval: a time lag of about 0.20 sec normally, caused by the time needed for transmission in the atrio-ventricular node and the atrio-ventricular bundle.

QRS complex: represents ventricular contraction (excitation or depolarisation). The right and left halves of the heart function almost synchronously.

T wave: represents relaxation of the ventricle (repolarisation).

From the *T* wave until the following *Q* wave the ventricles remain in the relaxed or polarised state.

The types of ECG to be found in association with the various pathological conditions will not be discussed.

It should be borne in mind that the electrical phenomena are not identical with the mechanical processes. Depolarisation initiates contraction. The coupling of the two processes is a field of study in itself with which we shall not deal here.

CHAPTER 4

EINTHOVEN'S TRIANGLE

In this chapter and the following one we shall present some fundamental conceptions which are basic in vectorcardiography. First we shall pay attention to the medical point of view and then, in Chapter 5, some basic formulae of electromagnetic theory will be considered.

4.1 The equilateral triangle

We start with a train of conceptions that originates with Einthoven [1]), a set of ideas which in spite of limitations and deficiences — which Einthoven himself fully recognized — had attracted much attention and which can be regarded as the basis of modern vectorcardiography.

Einthoven's reasoning ran more or less like this: given, that we overlook the fact that the heart is not located exactly in the middle of the body, let us further assume that the human body is completely symmetrical (inside and out), and finally let us assume that we can represent the electric activity of the heart as a directional value (Fig. 8) — designated by Einthoven as *"manifest potential difference"* or *"manifest value"*, and subsequently designated *"heart vector"*. (Some years later, as we shall still see, this representation is funded by the dipole conception.) If now, at a specific instant, this vector is directed along the long axis of the body, there would be no difference of potential between the right and left arm. When, on the contrary, the vector makes an angle with "the vertical", then the horizontal component of one of the two arms would be positive with respect to the other.

This concept which yields a relation between the magnitude and direction of the electric activity of the heart and the difference in potential between two points on the body (for a specific moment!) can be generalized. Einthoven accomplished this by means of an equilateral triangle, of which one of the sides was represented by the connecting line RL between right and

---

[1]) Einthoven performed pioneer work in the field of electrocardiography, his achievement being crowned by the Nobel price (1924). The uniformity that he brought into the discipline also testifies to his importance. We may mention here: sensitivity 1 millivolt $\sim$ 10 mm, page 4, speed of travel of the paper 25 mm/sec, page 5, localising of the electrodes on the extremities (page 11) and the expressions P, Q, R, S and T in the ECG (page 14).

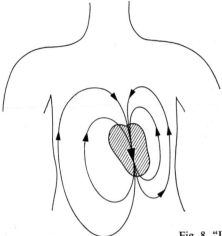

Fig. 8. "Instantaneous picture" of the heart vector

left arm, while the third angle of which was below the lower back or, if desired, at the usual location for the foot electrode (Fig. 9). The projections of the "arrow" on the three sides of this "Einthoven triangle" could then be taken approximately to represent the difference of potentional between the extremities (Fig. 10).

The idea gained general acceptance because of the simple and striking relationship between the limb leads and what could be conceived of the

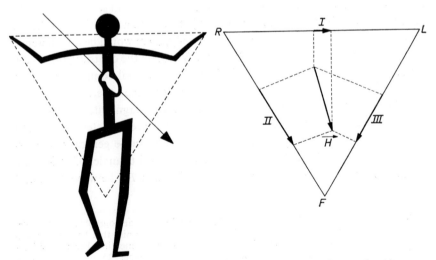

Fig. 9. Einthoven's equilateral triangle

Fig. 10. Projections of *H* on the sides of the triangle are of course not vectors!

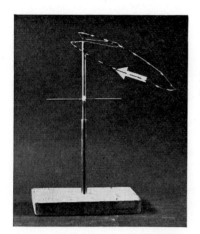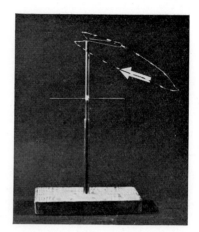

Fig. 13. Stereoscopic representation of the three-dimensional curve

(see text on page 21)

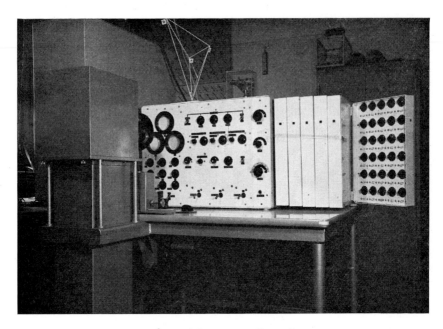

Fig. 26. The vectorcardiograph

(see text on page 42)

activity of the heart. Later we shall see that acceptance of the idea in this special form cannot be sustained. Even at this stage, we cite an argument that seemed to be of extreme importance at the time:

A proposition from plane geometry states that if the projections of a line on the sides of an equilateral triangle, furnished with the appropriate sign, are added, the sum is zero. A more elegant proof of the exactness of Eint- hoven's insight would be hard to find, because if we apply this proposition we have complete agreement with the rule that the sum of the differences of potential between R, L and F must be exactly zero (page 11)! Proceeding from subsequent observations, we already see how this dummy argument weakens when we consider that in fact the heart is not geometrically at the centre of the body, nor is the body symmetrical, and that moreover there is no valid reason for making the sides of the triangle exactly alike. A glance at Fig. 9 convinces us of the unreality of the notion that the association between heart vector and leads depends upon the length of the arms!

Einthoven's concept developed along various lines, sometimes in error. Because this development has led us step by step to present-day vectorcardio- graphy we shall mention some instances from the past in more detail.

In the first place there is the adaptation of instruments. The two-dimen- sional surface on which the heart vector H is assumed to move, made it possible to determine it directly from leads I, II and III. A simple calculation from plane geometry shows that the y-component H_y (a system of coordina- tes is introduced as in Fig. 11) to be determined is expressed as

$$y = \frac{2}{\sqrt{3}}\left(V_F - \frac{V_R + V_L}{2}\right). \qquad (4.1)$$

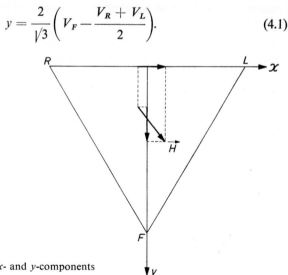

Fig. 11. Determination of x- and y-components of the heart vector H

while the x-component is simply represented by $V_L - V_R$. In other words, if the electrodes R and L are connected to a point Q via like resistors, the difference of potential between F and Q immediately yields the y-component in the form of a voltage, leaving out a factor $2/\sqrt{3}$ (which of course is easily to introduce in electronics).

If this voltage is connected to one pair of plates of a cathode ray tube and $V_L - V_R$ is connected to the other pair, then during a heart cycle a curve can be described which corresponds to the twodimensional course which the point of the arrow (representing the heart vector) traces. By periodic depression of the electron beam, a time marking can be introduced (see page 23). In this way, many years ago, a kind of vectorcardiogram could be recorded.

How far the acceptance of the conception of the triangle, which is in itself valuable, can lead in the direction of absurdity is illustrated by the fact that a cathode ray tube has been constructed with three paired plates at angles of 60°, to make a VCG directly from leads *I*, *II* and *III*. This no doubt expensive apparatus was apparently preferred to the use of a couple of resistors and an ordinary tube.

4.2 The equilateral tetrahedron

The abandonment of the flat surface, some years later, was a great step forward. With addition of a fourth electrode, e.g. on the back (*W*), the Einthoven triangle could be expanded to an equilateral tetrahedron (Wilson) (Fig. 12).

Here also, mistakenly, the assumption was that the projection of the heart vector on one of the ribs would yield the difference of potential between the

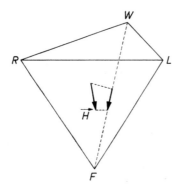

Fig. 12. Equilateral tetrahedron
W = Wilson

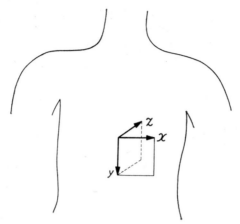

Fig. 14. System of coordinates in the human body. It must be noted that the directions of the axes have not been standardized

electrodes, coinciding with the angular points connected by that rib. However that may be, the idea that the electric heart activity was not a two-dimensional but rather a three-dimensional phenomenon was accepted. When represented by the heart vector this meant that "the arrow point" had not to describe a flat, but a three-dimensional curve (Fig. 13 opposite page 18). It was obvious that to determine this curve the heart vector had to be projected on three mutually perpendicular surfaces. For these there were chosen the *frontal*, the *horizontal* and the *sagittal* surfaces or respectively the X,Y, the X,Z and the Y,Z surfaces (Fig. 14). In practice this implies the determination of each of the components X, Y and Z of the heart vector H as a function of time from the differences of potential measured on the body surface. By this means each of the three projections (Fig. 15) can then be thrown on an oscilloscope screen and photographically recorded.

4.3 Cubic systems

Originally the attempt was made to select the locations of the electrodes in such a way that each pair separately would yield *one* component directly. It is clear that, even if such a localization (a so-called cubic system) exists it is in the nature of things that it will be hard to find it. Opinions on the matter were very divided, and at that moment the chaos concerning the field of vectorcardiography was born.

We will not review all the endeavours to place the electrodes in such a way that there would be no calculations to handle and the components of

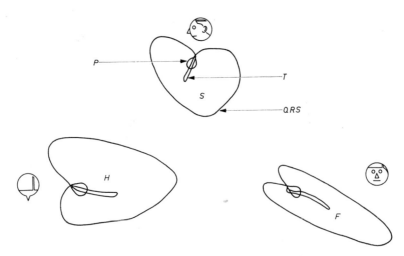

Fig. 15. A VCG (see also Fig. 73, page 125)
F. Frontal projection (x, y); *H.* horizontal projection (x, z); *S.* sagittal projection $(y, z$

the heart vector could be measured directly on the body surface. Systems thus developed were doomed to failure, certainly when they were based on intuition and not on physics.

It should be noted that in the course of years many systems were conceived some of which are still in use, which all produce data for use in their own way. Unfortunately, the vectorcardiograms based on the different systems are hardly comparable one with another and in fact a deplorable confusion has resulted.

4.4 General remarks on vectorcardiography

This poses the question, as to whether it is worthwhile to working towards physical development of vectorcardiography in the hope of achieving some uniformity in the future. It seems well at this point to probe the matter somewhat more deeply.

We might start with some pro-vectorcardiography arguments.

1. Vectorcardiography yields more information than electrocardiography. At first glance this seems to be a false premise since just as in electro-cardiography, differences of potential are measured on the body surface in vectorcardiography. And why should a combination of leads impart

more information than the individual leads? Of course, such a statement cannot hold, but there is, however, a fundamental difference in the way in which the two methods apply the information! While it is customary in electrocardiography to record the leads in succession, this recording is of necessity simultaneous in vectorcardiography so that a VCG essentially reflects phase differences. That these phases also contain information can be illustrated by the fact that in some cases a diagnosis can be made which is based exclusively on the phase difference (we will return to this) (page 132). It is true that often in electrocardiography also a number of leads are registered simultaneously but there is still uncertainty concerning the phase, since no single instrument is 100 percent reliable with respect to its time shift. For that matter, it is possible to extract only little information from them because the time resolution is too small.

An advantage which is of course not essential but which is nonetheless desirable is the way the information is achieved, namely that in vectorcardiography it is customary to work with somewhat greater sensitivity.

2a. Information is obtained in a more congenial form in many respects. In judging vectorcardiograms (Fig. 15) we use to a considerable degree our everyday ability to interpret certain shapes. We recognize our colleague instantly; the difference between a circle and an ellipse is immediately appreciated. We make use of this faculty in reading electrocardiograms too, although practical experience indicates that the reading is learned with more difficulty and more rapidly forgotten.

b. The total electric event during an entire heart cycle is reproduced and recorded by the closed circuit which is described by the dot on the oscilloscope screen. The electrocardiogram is "rolled up" as it were, so that the datum occupies a minimum of space.

c. The vectorcardiogram corresponds more closely to actual anatomy than does the ECG. The transmission of electricity and the position of the heart are simple concepts that we can imagine, and that we recover in the clear arrangement of the record. It is conceivable that we feel more at home in this case than with the specific physical method of reproduction of a magnitude that varies in time, whereby every direct correlation with reality is lacking, as is the case with the electrocardiogram.

For the sake of fairness, some drawbacks must also be noted. In the first place, the time element is practically eliminated in a vectorcardiogram. The deficiency is partially overcome by depression of the electron beam of the oscilloscope at constant known time intervals, so that a punctate image appears on the screen. From the record it is now possible to get an impression of the speed of advance (see Fig. 13) of the dot in each phase of the heart beat. The intensity of the dot does not drop abruptly, but rather it gradually diminishes, so that at the end of each strip a point appears (►) from which the direction of travel, which can be of great interest, can be determined (see Fig. 55, page 95) [1]). It is also sometimes difficult to see the transition from S- to T-loop in a vectorcardiogram (the so-called S-T segment).

Finally there is the intricate mathematical formulation which sometimes arouses resistance in the medical world.

If this barrier can be penetrated, vectorcardiography is surely a step in the right direction, toward as complete a knowledge as is possible of the electric behaviour of the human heart.

---

[1]) On this point the European convention does not agree with the American technique: In the European VCG's the arrow head indicates the forward direction of the dot motion; in American records the reverse is the case.

CHAPTER 5

THE ELECTRIC DIPOLE

5.1 Introduction

At the time when physics was first studied in relation to electrocardiography a large proportion of the appropriate theoretical work was clear. Before the application of this work can be understood certain concepts of electromagnetic theory must be examined. Of prime importance is the study of the dipole, understanding of which is essential in vectorcardiography.

When we study the way in which the physicist describes the phenomena which occur when a current passes through a medium we immediately encounter Ohm's law. If we omit complexities such as polarisation which are not essential for present purposes this law may be taken to apply also to the electrolytic conduction which takes place in the human body.

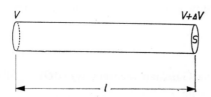

Fig. 16. Cylindrical piece of tissue

Let us assume, by analogy with a wire of conducting material, the existence of a homogeneous isotropic piece of tissue in the form of a small cylinder (Fig. 16) between the ends of which there is a difference of potential ΔV. The current passing through this cylinder may then be written thus:

$$L = \frac{\Delta V}{R} \tag{5.1}$$

Or, with $R = l/\sigma s$ in which σ is the specific conductivity, s the cross-sectional area and l the length of the cylinder:

$$I = \frac{\Delta V \sigma s}{l}. \tag{5.2}$$

For the current density j (= current per surface unit) we have

$$j = \frac{I}{s} = \frac{\Delta V \sigma}{l} = \sigma E \tag{5.3}$$

where E is the electrical field strength.

The expression thus obtained lends itself very well to generalisation and thus is useful in the consideration of other problems where we are not dealing with homogeneous potential fields such as the one discussed above. Thus, let E, σ and hence j be functions of the rectangular coordinates x, y and z. The expression for current density then becomes a vector equation which, when we limit ourselves to isotropic media — in which $\sigma(x,y,z)$ is a scalar — can be written thus

$$j = \sigma E \tag{5.4}$$

Naturally, the human body with its many different kinds of tissues is not isotropic but we will ignore the complications that this produces.

If we now consider an infinitesimal volume of tissue $dx\,dy\,dz$ as much electric charge will flow out as goes in (stationary current) or, expressed by formula

$$\int (j \cdot dO) = 0. \tag{5.5}$$

With reference to the Gaussian theorem $\int (j \cdot dO) = \int \text{div}\,j \cdot dV$ (here V is a volume) we may write

$$\text{div}\,j = \frac{\partial j_x}{\partial x} + \frac{\partial j_y}{\partial y} + \frac{\partial j_z}{\partial z} = 0 \tag{5.6}$$

In combination with the known relationship:

$$E = - \,\text{grad}\,V = -\left(\frac{\partial V}{\partial x}, \frac{\partial V}{\partial y}, \frac{\partial V}{\partial z}\right) = -\nabla V \tag{5.7}$$

and we obtain for div j (for a homogeneous medium)

$$\text{div}\,j = -\sigma\,\text{div}\,\text{grad}\,V = -\,\sigma\left(\frac{\partial^2 V}{\partial x^2} + \frac{\partial^2 V}{\partial y^2} + \frac{\partial^2 V}{\partial z^2}\right) = -\sigma\nabla^2 V = 0 \tag{5.8}$$

We obtain the important relationship

$$\nabla^2 V = 0 \text{ (Laplace equation).} \tag{5.9}$$

What formalism can we now derive for an element of the myocardium itself?

Since the electrical phenomena originate at this point, these phenomena have to be recovered in the description with local quantities. Clearly, a single extra term in the expression for j represents the difference between the current density in a volume element inside the heart and that in an element outside the heart. If we designate the electromotive field strength, caused by the heart action, E^* and the electromotive current density j^* then

$$\text{outside the heart} \quad j = \sigma E = -\sigma \nabla V \qquad (5.10)$$

$$\text{inside the heart} \quad j = \sigma E + \sigma E^* = -\sigma \nabla V + j^* \qquad (5.11)$$

In both cases: div $j = 0$.

The extra term $\sigma E^* \equiv j^*$ for the myocardium is essential to electrocardiography. It precisely characterises the electrical action of the heart produced by electrolytical processes in the muscle tissue. The determination of this E^* as a function of place and time will yield information concerning the normal or abnormal functioning of the heart. It must be immediately added that this quantity cannot be determined from measurements of potential differences on the body surface; however the attempt can be made to determine it as far as possible (see also page 67).

Having derived the above information we shall penetrate further into some pure physics and later, armed with the knowledge thus obtained, we shall return to the study of the heart.

Let us consider a homogeneous isotropic and infinitely extended medium to which, at a point P, a current I is applied (e.g. with a long wire which is insulated, except at the outer end) and again taken off at infinity (a so-called single pole, Fig. 17). Note first that the currents spreads from the point of

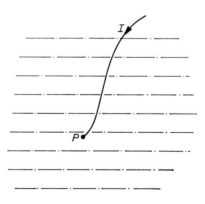

Fig. 17. Single pole

introduction with spherical symmetry. The current density at distance r from P is then

$$j_r = \frac{I}{4\pi r^2} \qquad (5.12)$$

or, with $j_r = \sigma E_r$

$$j_r = \sigma E_r = -\sigma \frac{dV}{dr} = \frac{I}{4\pi r^2} \qquad (5.13)$$

If we integrate (5.13) with boundary condition $V_\infty = 0$, then for the potential at distance r from P we have

$$V = \frac{I}{4\pi\sigma r} \qquad (5.14)$$

5.2 The electric dipole

Let us now imagine not one but two wires inserted in the medium, one of which supplies the current while the other carries it off, or in other words two poles, one positive and one negative — a so-called *current doublet* — and then consider the question of the potentional at an arbitrary point Q (Fig. 18). We assign the point Q by the distance r measured from the middle of the connecting line δ between the two poles and by the angle θ which r makes with δ. We obtain V by superposition of the potentials produced by each of the two poles separately, thus:

$$V = \frac{I}{4\pi\sigma} \left(\frac{1}{r_{(+)}} - \frac{1}{r_{(-)}} \right) \qquad (5.15)$$

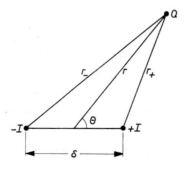

Fig. 18. Current doublet

If we make $\delta \ll r$, the above formula becomes

$$V = \frac{I\delta \cos \theta}{4\pi\sigma r^2} \tag{5.16}$$

We now let $\delta \to 0$ and at the same time let I increase in such a manner that the product $I\delta \equiv D_i$ remains constant. Then, in the limit, we obtain a *dipole* and we can describe the field thus:

$$V = \frac{D_i \cos \theta}{4\pi\sigma r^2} \tag{5.17}$$

We shall see over and over again what an important place the concept of the dipole occupies in the description of the electrical phenomena in the heart. For this reason we shall discuss this concept more fully and approach the problem from two further angles.

5.3 Examples

Imagine a spherical part of a homogeneous infinitely extended conducting medium. Inside this part we assume an arbitrary number of poles to be present, both positive and negative, so that we know the currents that come into the medium and leave it, as well as the coordinates of each pole, in a polar coordinates system, of which the origin is situated in the middle of the sphere. Once again we study the potential V at a point Q outside the sphere, at a distance r from the centre (Fig. 19). In principle we can of course obtain V by summing the potentials at each pole separately. However nothing essentially new emerges from such a calculation. It is more profitable to try to develop V in a power series in r (see also page 110).

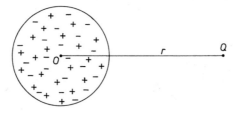

Fig. 19. Current poles in a conducting medium

Since the choice of an infinitely extended medium also permits $r = \infty$ and anyhow the series must converge, only negative powers of r are allowed. Thus we may write:

$$V = \frac{\Phi_1}{r} + \frac{\Phi_2}{r^2} + \frac{\Phi_3}{r^3} + \ldots + \frac{\Phi_i}{r^i} + \ldots \tag{5.18}$$

(only valid outside the sphere!) wherein Φ_i is a function of the direction of the radius vector at Q and must have such a form that $\nabla^2 V = 0$ (see Chapter 14, p. 103). Remember that the field of a single pole is described by $V = I/4\pi\sigma r$. From this we can conclude that the first term is none other than the potential of the total single pole formed by all poles together. Since V must satisfy the Laplace equation $\nabla^2 V = 0$ and, moreover, since we assumed that on the whole no current goes in or out of the sphere, this term in our case equals zero. By analogy we see that the second term represents the potential of the total dipole while the subsequent terms represent poles of higher orders. For this representation to be applicable in practice it is naturally necessary for the series to converge rapidly.

Finally, we shall consider a simple and completely calculable case. We shall take a homogeneous conducting and infinitely extended space. In a spherical part thereof (radius a) there is a known constant homogeneous electromotive field strength E^* acting in direction x (Fig. 20). (The coordinate system is assumed to be the same as under (a).) That part of the space inside the sphere we shall designate 1 and that part outside will be called 2. By analogy with what has been said above (page 27)

$$j = -\sigma\nabla V + \sigma E^* \tag{5.11}$$

is valid,
with $E^* = $ constant for $r \ll a$
and $E^* = 0$ for $r > a$
and div $j = 0$ for all r, with boundary condition for $r = a$.

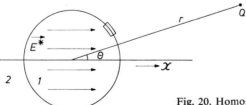

Fig. 20. Homogeneous electromotive field strength

We should now find an expression for V_1 and V_2, both as functions of r and θ. For V_1 we expect an equation with a positive power of r because within the sphere the potential must remain finite, while in the formula for V_2, r will appear with a negative power, that for r_∞, $V \to 0$. Moreover in both cases $\nabla^2 V = 0$ must be satisfied. It appears then that:

$$V_1 = Ar \cos \theta = Ax \qquad (5.19)$$

and

$$V_2 = \frac{B \cos \theta}{r^2} \qquad (5.20)$$

wherein A and B are constants, i.e., independent of the coordinates r and θ. Equations (5.19) and (5.20) (the latter of which represents a dipole effect) will be justified in the following calculation.

We can determine A and B by means of the boundary conditions:

a. The potential at the surface of the sphere ($r = a$) must be continuous, i.e. we must be able to describe V with the equation for V_2 as well as with that for V_1. Since the potential must have a unique value,

$$Aa \cos \theta = B \frac{\cos \theta}{a^2}$$

from which it follows that

$$B = a^3 A \qquad (5.21)$$

b. For the second boundary condition we shall consider a thin box-shaped element located half in the sphere and half in space 2 (see Fig. 20). For this element the entering current is the same as the outgoing current (div $j = 0$), thus the normal component of the current density calculated from 1 and also from 2, must yield the same result. So we obtain a second relationship between A and B:

$$-\sigma \operatorname{grad} V_1 + \sigma E^* \cos \theta = -\sigma \operatorname{grad} V_2$$

or

$$-A\sigma \cos \theta + \sigma E^* \cos \theta = 2 B\sigma \frac{\cos \theta}{a^3} . \qquad (5.22)$$

Combination of (5.21) and (5.22) yields for V_2:

$$V_2 = \frac{E^* \cos \theta\, a^3}{3r^2} = \frac{E^* 4/3 \cdot \pi a^3 \cos \theta}{4/3 \cdot \pi\, 3r^2}$$

hence:

$$V_2 = \frac{E^* \cdot \text{volume} \cdot \cos \theta}{4\pi r^2} \tag{5.23}$$

If we now write $E^* \cdot \text{volume} = D_v$ and $D_v = D_i/\sigma$, we get exactly the expression that we calculated for the potential as a result of a *current* dipole (page 29, (5.17)).

(5.23) is the expression for a *voltage* dipole.

From this simplified picture it appears that the terms of higher order in the general series progression (see *a*) are lacking here.

Finally let us assume that E^* is a function of the coordinates. Then evidently (5.23) goes over into an integral form:

$$V_2 = \frac{\underset{\text{vol}}{\int} E^*(\mathbf{r}) \cos \theta \, d(\text{vol})}{4\pi r^2} \tag{5.24}$$

Here the form of the volume is arbitrary.

CHAPTER 6

THE RELATIONSHIP BETWEEN HEART VECTOR AND LEADS. THE VECTORCARDIOGRAPH

After considering the advances in medicine and physics, which had been developed separately, we shall now attempt to link the two.

In the trunk the electric current satisfies a differential equation (Chapter 5), thereby we have boundary conditions for the body surface and for the immediate vicinity of the source of electricity. It is thus clear that, with an exact physical treatment of what occurs in the human body with reference to electric activity of the heart, we confront a complicated problem as so often in biophysics. A simplification is in order.

1. *Linearity*

All phenomena of which we attempt to discover the background are *linear*. This is suggested by an equation such as div $j = 0$ (see 5.6), an equation of the first order, thus without products or squares, and by the linear relationship between current density and field strength (Ohm's law) or by the boundary condition $j_n = 0$. We will make use of this linearity right up to the end.

2. *Dipole approximation*

We assume all electric phenomena to be caused by a dipole which is stationary with respect to place (for definition of the dipole see page 29). This approximation will only be applied provisionally. In Chapter 10 we shall come to a more rigorous treatment. (We use the expression *"dipole approximation"* where others use *"dipole hypothesis"*. Since the word "hypothesis" is out of place here, we depart from usual terminology.)

In principle there are three methods to describe the relationship between the heart vector and the observed phenomena:

6.1 Analytic approach

We select a simple problem, by representing the human body as a homogeneous isotropic medium with a spherical outline. If we assume the dipole of the heart to be in the center thereof, we can calculate without difficulty the distribution of potential on the surface (Chapter 5). Vice versa, we can derive some knowledge of the source from study of this distribution of potential. (Note however what is said about this on page 27 and 67.)

If we postulate more complicated conditions, we can extend our formalism. By this means we can gain some insight into the material but it is clear that little can be expected from this in practice, since the actual problem is too complex.

6.2 The digital method

We can attempt to solve the differential equation with limiting conditions by numerical calculation. The subject will however not be treated in this book.

6.3 The analogue method. Model experiments

Here we make use of a model: a system that simulates as accurately as possible the subject we are investigating. In this model we can now choose or vary a number of magnitudes (actually an unknown number) in order to be able to follow by measurement their effects upon our model system. The knowledge gained in this way can then later be applied to the solution of the actual problem.

In our case the model will be a more or less accurate copy of the human body: a cavity filled with an electrolyte, having an artificial heart.

What we will measure is the distribution of potential over the surface as a function of magnitude and direction of the heart vector. Following our working approximation, we use for our artificial heart an electric doublet (thereby approximating the dipole) which is so constructed (we shall come back to this subject on page 38) that orientation and pole strength can be suitably chosen.

Before we go into practical details, we will first formulate the problem in greater detail, in the solution of which the model can help us.

If we assign the three components of the heart vector (in our model the dipole vector) as $X(t)$, $Y(t)$ and $Z(t)$, then because of the linear relationship, (page 33) we may write for the difference of potential between any two electrodes P and P_0.

$$V_P - V_{P_0} = a(\xi, \eta)X(t) + b(\xi, \eta)Y(t) + c(\xi, \eta)Z(t) = V(\xi, \eta, t). \qquad (6.1)$$

Here a, b and c are "constants" dependent only on the location of P (expressed in the arbitrary body coordinates ξ and η) and *not on time*; P_0 is assumed to be a fixed reference point. This expression which gives us the relationship between one specific lead and the heart vector with its three time-dependent components and which is valid independently of the properties of the model, can also be generally stated:

$$V(\xi, \eta, t) = c_1(\xi, \eta) f_1(t) + c_2(\xi, \eta) f_2(t) + c_3(\xi, \eta) f_3(t) + c_4(\xi, \eta) f_4(t) + \ldots$$
$$(6.2)$$

Thus a linear combination of a plurality of time functions. The dipole approximation permits us to break off the series behind the third term since the dipole vector has only three components. For a more exact description however, as shown later (Chapter 14), we shall need to use higher terms.

For each of the ∞^2 electrocardiograms that we can make for one subject, an equation of this kind can be written. Let us restrict ourselves to the minimum of three (independent) leads, we then get three equations of this kind, e.g. (in simplified notation)

$$V_{P_1} - V_{P_0} = V_1 = a_1 X + b_1 Y + c_1 Z$$
$$V_{P_2} - V_{P_0} = V_2 = a_2 X + b_2 Y + c_2 Z \qquad (6.3)$$
$$V_{P_3} - V_{P_0} = V_3 = a_3 X + b_3 Y + c_3 Z$$

If we could determine the nine constants a_i, b_i and c_i then we could solve for X, Y and Z at any moment of the heart cycle from the potential differences, since the three components of the heart vector must satisfy:

$$X = \alpha_1 V_1 + \alpha_2 V_2 + \alpha_3 V_3$$
$$Y = \beta_1 V_1 + \beta_2 V_2 + \beta_3 V_3 \qquad (6.4)$$
$$Z = \gamma_1 V_1 + \gamma_2 V_2 + \gamma_3 V_3$$

in which α_j, β_j and γ_j are known functions of a_i, b_i and c_i. In other words we could calculate the behaviour of the heart vector during an entire heart cycle [1]).

At this stage the model is of use: it offers us the possibility of finding the coefficients a_i, b_i and c_i by approximation. For this we orientate the artificial heart so that the dipole vector is directed along one of the axes of the coordinate system that we have assumed in the body or in the model (see fig. 14, page 21).

If we select for this direction the x-axis, then the y- and z-component of

---

[1]) As known, three equations with three unknowns are only soluble as the determinant $|\alpha_j \beta_j \gamma_j| \neq 0$. In practice this means that the said determinant must not be too small.

the dipole vector will be zero and the set of equations (6.4) will be reduced to

$$V_i = a_i X. \tag{6.5}$$

We can calculate a_i from this since V_i is derived directly from a measurement and X can be chosen arbitrarily by ourselves, at least to a relative value. Analogously we determine values for b_i and c_i by orientating the dipole vector along the y- and z-axis respectively.

The fact that the coefficients a_i, b_i and c_i are dependent upon the locations of the electrodes implies that the properties of the model are of major importance. Care must therefore be taken in construction of the phantom. Without entering into details we shall make a few remarks on this subject with special reference to the model used in the laboratory in Utrecht (Fig. 21).

"Michaplast" (insulating material) is used to make a hollow form of a man lying prone, 1/3 natural size. The interior is accessible through a slit parallel to the frontal plane. The artificial heart can be inserted through an aperture in the back. The cavity is filled with a copper sulphate solution. Evidently it is not possible to simulate all the natural inhomogeneities, and we can do no more than take into account some very poorly conducting

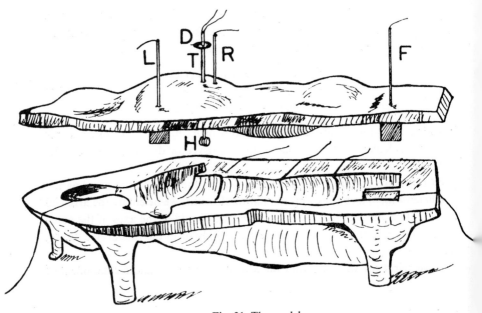

Fig. 21. The model
A: chest-side; *B*: back-side; *L*, *R* and *F*: extremity electrodes; *H*: artificial heart; *T*: glass tube; *D*: dial

parts in the immediate vicinity of the heart, for example the vertebral column and the lungs.

Obviously all these arrangements cannot be made arbitrarily, but rather they must be based on measurements made on the human body. Without going into the technicalities of measurement, we simply note that for the specific conductivity of "normal" muscle tissue a value of 200 to 300 $\Omega \cdot cm$ (longitudinal measurement) was determined, and that bone is a very poor conductor, while for the specific resistance of the lungs a magnitude approximately four times that of the surrounding tissue was assumed. In the model we used a cork spinal column. The lungs appeared to be simulated satisfactorily with two modelled sand bags.

Concerning the latter a few more remarks can be made. It is obvious that the ratio of resistance between "lungs" and electrolyte is independent of the concentration of the copper sulfate solution. Perhaps it is less obvious that the relationship is not affected by the absolute size of the grains of sand either. If the grains are larger, then the interstices between them are larger too and total conductivity remains unchanged. It is the law of *frequency distribution* that governs the way in which the space between the larger grains is filled up by the smaller ones.

How much the model still leaves to be desired in the way of authenticity is indicated by the fact that no account is taken of the important anisotropy of muscle tissue (a striated muscle has a much greater specific conductivity in the longitudinal direction than in the direction perpendicular thereto).

The model has neither arms nor legs. The electric current emanating from the heart hardly penetrates into these members so that — as already noted (page 11) — the extremities can be considered as equipotential volumes.

Since opinions concerning magnitude and effect of inhomogeneities in the body are not always unanimous, there is, in addition to the above described standpoint, still another with respect to phantom design. The premise is that a hollow form filled with electrolyte alone (hence no lungs etc.) also yields a meaningful approximation of reality — with or without realizing that there is a greater distortion of reality than necessary. According to the holders of this opinion, the object of the search can not be the dipole whereby the electric activity of the heart can best be characterized, but must rather be an *effective dipole*. An effective dipole is understood to be the dipole that we should establish for the homogeneous model, to bring measurements made thereon into conformity with those made on the human body.

With all the shortcoming inherent in these models, there is at hand the human body itself which may be used as a model, in other words — measurement on cadavers. However great the advantages may be, there are still many sources of error, among them those that stem from postmortem changes. We note only that many experiments have been done in this area, not always unsuccessfully.

A few remarks may be made with reference to the artificial heart, the dipole generator.

Construction is as follows: two circular copper plates P_1 and P_2, each about 2 cm in diameter, are mounted on a cylinder 2 cm long, made of insulating material (Fig. 22). By means of 4-volts storage batteries a predetermined difference of potential can be established between the two plates (voltage dipole). A current will then flow in the liquid along lines of conducting as shown in the figure.

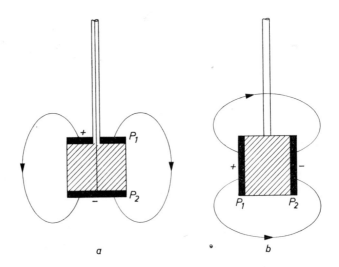

Fig. 22. Two possible forms of the artificial heart

The dipole of Fig. 22a only permits an orientation in the y direction, the artificial heart of Fig. 22b makes x and z directions accessible. Use is simpler in the embodiment of Fig. 23. The poles here are attached on the six surfaces of a cube oriented along the coordinate system. Component X, Y or Z can easily be selected by connecting the voltage source to the appropriate wires.

The question may be asked, what kind of dipole should be selected for the generator. There are three kinds: load, current and voltage dipole. It should be evident that the first type cannot be used for practical purposes, since in

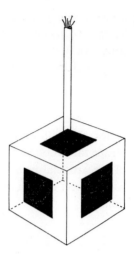

Fig. 23. An artificial heart of which the x, y or z component can easily be selected

a conducting medium such as an electrolyte it is impossible to provide the conductor with a charge which can be applied as desired. The choice between voltage and current dipole remains. If we restrict ourselves to relative values then it appears that the two types are quite identical.

Up to the present, measurements of a_i, b_i and c_i have always been relative measurements. Evidently it is possible to assign absolute values, by determining absolute values for V_i and X in the equation:

$$V_i = a_i X \qquad (6.5)$$

V_i can naturally be read directly from a voltmeter, but X must be determined by calculation. Concerning the latter we recall what was said above with respect to the mathematical expression for the dipole (Chapter 5).

If we take a voltage dipole as our starting point, the potential V at a point Q at distance r (apart from a constant) satisfies

$$V = \frac{D_v \cos \theta}{4\pi r^2} \qquad (6.6)$$

(see also 5.17 page 29 and page 31). This expression is only valid, as we mentioned elsewhere (page 29) for a pure dipole (mutual distances of the poles $\rightarrow 0$, pole strength $\rightarrow \infty$ and $D_v =$ constant). If in practice we attempt to approximate this ideal, we must apply a very high voltage between the smallest possible poles. But then such great current densities will be developed in the immediate vicinity of the poles that numerous complications will arise, for example heating the electrolyte and consequent local lessening of the specific resistance. For this reason we prefer a doublet for our articifial heart: two metallic plates (diameter $2a$) mutually separated by distance d (Fig. 24). The expression for the dipole moment of such a system, already calculated by Maxwell, reads

$$D_v = \Delta V \pi a^2 f\,(d/a)\ \text{volt·m}^2 \tag{6.7}$$

(This expression is only valid if there is no insulating material between the plates. We will not discuss in detail the known form of f in this equation). Hence the absolute magnitude of the dipole vector, or of the "heart vector" of the artificial heart used is determined. By making the plates adjustable with respect to each other, the size of the vector can be varied within certain limits.

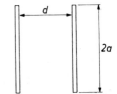

Fig. 24. According to Maxwell's formula

It should be noted that all this is reported only to show how *absolute* values for a, b and c may be obtained. In practice only *relative* values are used. In vectorcardiography it is above all the form of the spatial curve that is considered to be important rather than absolute size. It is true that occasionally work has been done on relative size [1] but clinically it is not very important.

6.4 The vectorcardiograph

The association mentioned above between leads and heart vector is the natural basis of the instrumentation. We will consider it briefly.

The starting point of course is the three relationships (6.4) (page 35) where the three components $X(t)$, $Y(t)$ and $Z(t)$ of the heart vector yield as *linear combination* of the used leads $V_i(t)$:

---

[1] For normal use, work is performed with a standard apparatus sensitivity. If the loop for an individual patient is so large that it is no longer shown completely on the screen, the sensitivity can be reduced to say 0.7 of normal.

$$X(t) = \alpha_1 V_1(t) + \alpha_2 V_2(t) + \alpha_3 V_3(t)$$
$$Y(t) = \beta_1 V_1(t) + \beta_2 V_2(t) + \beta_3 V_3(t) \qquad (6.4)$$
$$Z(t) = \gamma_1 V_1(t) + \gamma_2 V_2(t) + \gamma_3 V_3(t).$$

On the preceding pages (page 35 and up) we explained how magnitudes $\alpha_1 \ldots \gamma_3$ could be determined with the aid of model experiments. We shall assume these 9 coefficients to be known in the following.

It is clear — we already indicated it (page 21) — that voltages $X(t)$, $Y(t)$ and $Z(t)$ when they are accurately applied to the deflecting plates of oscilloscopes, make it possible for us to make the three projections of the vector-cardiogram visible. We shall discuss how we can realize this experimentally.

As an example, let us assume that the three independent leads V_1, V_2 and V_3 correspond to the potential differences which are found between four electrodes for which we select the previously mentioned three limb electrodes R, L, F and a fourth B, on the chest. With this in mind we rewrite (6.4) (it appears to be a practical advantage to take the electrode on the right arm as the point of reference):

$$X = \alpha_1(V_L - V_R) + \alpha_2(V_F - V_R) + \alpha_3(V_B - V_R)$$
$$Y = \beta_1(V_L - V_R) + \beta_2(V_F - V_R) + \beta_3(V_B - V_R) \qquad (6.8)$$
$$Z = \gamma_1(V_L - V_R) + \gamma_2(V_F - V_R) + \gamma_3(V_B - V_R)$$

What is to be done by the vectorcardiograph is the adding of voltages in such a way that each voltage is given its exact "weight factor".

We shall indicate two methods by which our object can be attained.

1. The first is a method which is frequently used, but which is not at all flexible. A circuit is established as sketched in Fig. 25, whereby in principle the above mentioned mathematical operation can be carried out. (Points L, F and B in Fig. 25 represent the corresponding electrodes.) With Ohm's and Kirchhoff's laws it is easy to verify that, if resistances r_L, r_F and r_B are large

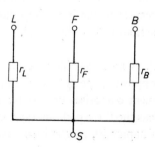

Fig. 25. Addition of voltages having the same sign

with respect to the internal resistance of system LFB, the difference of potential between point S and any other point (in our case electrode R) is the weighted average of voltages L, F and B each with that point. Thus, with $\sigma_i = 1/r_i$

$$V_S = c(\sigma_L V_L + \sigma_F V_F + \sigma_B V_B) \qquad (6.9)$$

wherein the constant $c = 1/(\sigma_L + \sigma_F + \sigma_B)$. (It seems sometimes to be handier in mathematical technique to work with the conductivity σ instead of with the resistance r.) Applying (6.9) the x-component from (6.4) becomes:

$$X = V_S - V_R = C_x[\sigma_{Lx}(V_L - V_R) + \sigma_{Fx}(V_F - V_R) + \sigma_{Bx}(V_B - V_R)] \quad (6.10)$$

wherein $\sigma_{Lx} \sim \alpha_1$, $\sigma_{Fx} \sim \alpha_2$ and $\sigma_{Bx} \sim \alpha_3$ (we do not pay attention for a moment to the constant C_x which is not very important in vectorcardiography).

Analogue expressions hold for the y- and z-component of the heartvector.

Only voltages having the same sign can be added by this method. For the general case in which there are also negative coefficients, the method must be extended. For example use can be made of a differential amplifier at one grid of which positive voltages are applied via resistors, while to the other grid, also via resistors, the potential differences are applied, provided with a negative coefficient.

Unfortunately, if coefficients $\alpha_1 \ldots \gamma_3$ are to be realized by means of resistors, one system of vectorcardiography cannot be simply exchanged for another. This can be understood if we bear in mind that it is true that the absolute values of components X, Y and Z in vectorcardiography do not play an important part, but that obviously all components must be accorded *the same weight*, which is achieved by making C_y and C_z equal to C_x (electronically signified by introduction of an extra resistor). If now one coefficient is changed — thus one resistor — then the entire system of resistors must be adjusted to this change. If we also realize that all resistances in the system must be large in comparison to those in the electrode system and small with respect to the input impedance of the amplifier, then we see that this rigid system is less than ideal.

2. A more flexible method is applied in the vectorcardiograph (Fig. 26 see opposite page 40) as developed at Utrecht and still in use there. This instrument comprises two parts: a preamplifier and the apparatus proper, which has the three cathode ray tubes. The former has five different channels (later, Chapter 10, we shall see how we come to combining more than three inde-

pendent leads) each of which as a final stage has a cathode follower. Between each cathode follower and the succeeding differential amplifier, the voltage is divided with a potentiometer to a value that is proportional to the difference of potential between the input electrodes, multiplied by the appropriate coefficient. All voltages thus obtained from the five channels are delivered to the grids of differential amplifiers via like resistors. The buttons whereby the potentiometers are operated are on the righthand side of the apparatus (Fig. 26). The five columns correspond to the (maximally) five leads to be combined. The six rows correspond to the two deflecting devices of each of the three oscilloscopes. Below each potentiometer there is an additional small button whereby the sign (of the coefficient) can be selected.

Before use the instrument can be calibrated with the aid of an alternating current supply, producing 1 millivolt. A switch connects this signal with the various input electrodes. On each of the three oscilloscope screens there then appears a straight line whereon the correct components are given in horizontal and vertical direction by turning the knobs of the potentiometers.

The advantage of this method over the one previously described is *the simple manner in which the vectorcardiograph can be adapted to many systems of vectorcardiography*. Even in the instrument here described, six different systems (or transformations, see Chapter 11) may be realised at a time (see the six setting devices at the right) which can be connected to the cathode ray tube via a selector switch.

Moreover because of the low output impedance of the cathode follower there is more freedom of choice with respect to the magnitude of the resistances.

Finally we will indicate a few more general features of the instrument shown in Fig. 26: The three oscilloscope screens are photographed by means of a camera constructed especially for this purpose (Fig. 26, left). A so-called *beam depressor* is built into the apparatus to prevent the occurrence of great differences of blackening and to even excess radiation in the image as the result of the varying speeds at which the dot moves across the screen. This lessens the intensity of the electron beam at low speeds or at rest (diastolic interval). Finally, the vectorcardiograph has a device to produce a punctate image, as indicated on page 24.

CHAPTER 7

GEOMETRICAL REPRESENTATION

7.1 The lead vector

We return to the expression

$$V_P - V_{P_0} = V(\xi, \eta, t) = a(\xi, \eta)X(t) + b(\xi, \eta)Y(t) + c(\xi, \eta)Z(t) \qquad (6.1)$$

(see page 34) which describes the relationship between the heart vector and the difference of potential between two arbitrarily selected electrodes P and P_0 (see page 34 and 35). This equation is essentially a relationship between a *scalar* (V) and a vector (XYZ). A relationship of this kind can only be realized when the righthand member is the *scalar product of two vectors*! In other words we can also write (in simplified notation)

$$V = (abc \cdot XYZ) \qquad (7.1)$$

in which we designate abc the *lead vector*. We can also express this geometrically (Fig. 27). At any instant the difference of potential between P and P_0,

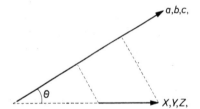

Fig. 27. Lead vector

can thus be determined by multiplying the projection of XYZ from that instant on the constant vector abc (determined by the location of P and P_0) by the absolute value of abc, or

$$V = |abc| \cdot |XYZ| \cdot \cos \theta$$

where θ is the included angle.

7.2 The lead triangle

Let us apply this to the three known limb leads (right arm, left arm and left leg). We know that the sum of the three voltages is zero

$$V_L - V_R = a_1X + b_1Y + c_1Z$$
$$V_R - V_F = a_2X + b_2Y + c_2Z$$
$$V_F - V_L = a_3X + b_3Y + c_3Z$$

$$\overline{} +$$

$$0 \quad = (a_1 + a_2 + a_3)X + \ldots . \tag{7.2}$$

If this is to be so, independent of time, then the following must be valid

$$a_1 + a_2 + a_3 = 0, \; b_1 + b_2 + b_3 = 0, \; c_1 + c_2 + c_3 = 0.$$

This is equivalent to the statement that the three lead vectors $a_1b_1c_1$, $a_2b_2c_2$ and $a_3b_3c_3$ must total zero when vectorally added, i.e., together they must constitute a triangle. If we now think of such a triangle with the heart vector drawn inside it (Fig. 28), then we can determine the difference of potential between the extremities at any instant by projecting the vector on the sides

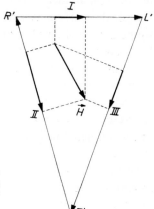

Fig. 28. Lead triangle $R'L'F'$. The primes are used so that angles of the triangle will not be confused with the locations of the electrodes R, L and F on the body

of the triangle and multiplying each projection by the length of the matching side (the absolute value of the lead vector).

We thus arrive at a conception analogous with that of Einthoven and obviously we make comparison between the two: Just as in the case of the equilateral triangle of Einthoven, here also the analytic formulation of the summing rule is proved by a theorem [1]) from plane geometry. The difference

---

[1]) If each projection from a line on the sides of a triangle is multiplied by the length of the matching side of the triangle, the sum of these products (provided with the correct signs) is zero.

however is that now the problem is physically based and that it is no longer essential that the triangle be equilateral.

It should be noted that it decidedly is not a necessity that the vector be placed in the triangle. It will be understood that nothing in the logical argument is changed if we separate arrow and triangle from each other, provided that the mutual directional positioning *is left unaltered*.

7.3 The image surface

Our proposition can now be generalized. Let us assume that we add a fourth electrode. There are then three different leads possible with R, L and F, namely each of these combined with the fourth. Each of these leads implies a lead vector, which is fixed in magnitude and direction. Bearing in mind that at each setting of three electrodes the above mentioned triangle rule is valid, we can form an idea of the spatial analogue of the lead triangle: It must be a tetrahedron. Here also we determine the difference of potential between two points (or electrodes) at a specific instant, by multiplying the length of the connecting side by the projection of the heart vector on that side.

Continuing our generalisation, we shall discover what happens with an arbitrary expansion of this number of four electrodes. If we take a fifth electrode and determine its lead vector, this in our spatial representation, e.g. extending from point R, will lead to a specific point in space. This point is then correlated with the location of the fifth electrode on the human body or model.

We proceed with a 6th, 7th, 8th ... ∞ electrode, producing the same amount of points in space. This develops what is called the *"image surface"*. In accordance with the above operation we can establish an *"image point"* on the image surface for any point on the body surface. (We must note that the introduction of the image surface is entirely based on the "dipole approximation" hence on the existence of the heart vector.)

7.4 Examples

In the following discussion we shall distinguish the location of the electrode and the image thereof in the image space by providing the latter with a prime. Thus R and R' etc. (In Fig. 28 we have already applied this notation.)

Using simple examples, we shall elucidate the geometric representation more closely.

7.4.1. We imagine a two-dimensional conductive layer with an arbitrary boundary (Fig. 29). Somewhere in the layer we asume the presence of a known stationary dipole [1]). If we select, finally, at some location e.g. on the periphery (the analogue of the surface of the human body) a zero point, then we can measure the potentials at any point on the periphery with reference to that zero point. For such a point k

$$V_k - V_0 = a_k X + b_k Y \qquad (7.3)$$

is valid. If we orient the dipole so that its vector is directed along the x-axis, the y-component is then zero, and

$$(V_k)_x - V_0 = a_k X. \qquad (7.4)$$

If we then make $X = 1$, then (7.4) becomes

$$(V_k)_x - V_0 = a_k. \qquad (7.5)$$

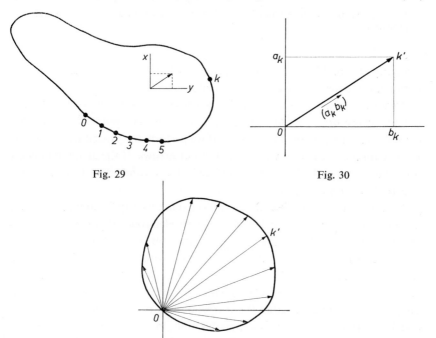

Fig. 29   Fig. 30

Fig. 31 Example of the construction of an image surface

---

[1]) In practice the layer will not be two-dimensional, but will have a finite thickness. In order to agree with the result of the experiment with the real two-dimensional case, the dipole is constructed as two parallel wires, placed perpendicularly on the layer, a so-called dipole line.

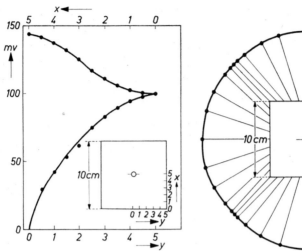

Fig. 32. Measured distribution of potential

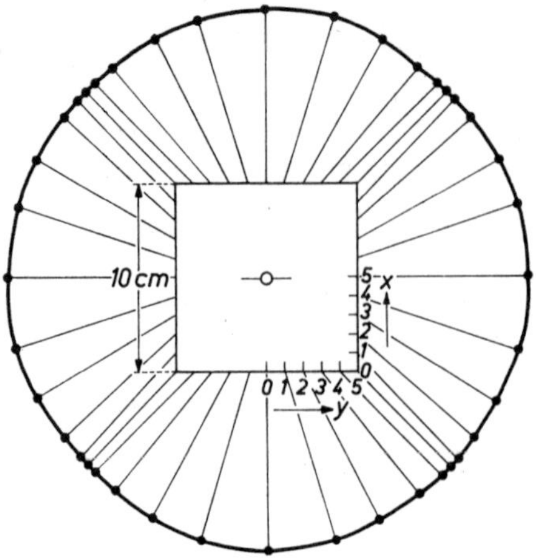

Fig. 33. Square with its image surface

Similarly, by making the dipole vector coincide with the y-axis, we may obtain a value for b_k. The two components of the lead vector are thus known, and we can construct $(a_k b_k)$. For this purpose we assume a system of coordinates whose origin is the representation of the zero point (V_0) (Fig. 30), chosen on the periphery of our object. If we perform the procedure for "each" point k on the periphery, we obtain a fan of arrows. If the arrow points are now interconnected, the "image surface" of the conductive layer appears. Figure 31 shows a schema thereof [1]).

A point on the image surface is established in this way for any point on the actual surface. The lead vector of a pair of electrodes (here thought of as being on the periphery of the conductive surface) is obtained by connecting the corresponding points of the image surface with each other. The correlation between the points of both surfaces must be known, of course. This correlation can be given most conveniently by drawing the object within the image surface and connecting the corresponding points by lines (see Fig. 33 and Fig. 34). (This is of course possible only in two-dimensional cases.) It must emphatically be noted that *these lines have no meaning* other than that which they have here for this particular purpose.

---

[1]) No particular value is to be attached to the form of this image surface (Fig. 31). The choice is arbitrary, neither based on actual measurements nor upon calculation.

7.4.2. The following example gives the result of an experiment. In a square tank filled with electrolyte, a dipole (better a dipole line; see foot note page 47) is placed so that the dipole vector is directed along the y-axis. The distribution of potential along the periphery of the tank with reference to an arbitrary zero point can be measured. Fig. 32 presents the result of these measurements for one quadrant of the square, whereby the point of reference is at the middle of one of the sides. Without going into details of the method, it can be seen that the image surface can be determined by it, in a manner similar to that described in paragraph 7.4.1. (For the sake of symmetry a separate measurement in the case of a dipole oriented along the x-axis can be omitted). Fig. 33 shows the image surface in which each point is correlated with a point on the square.

Just as we can *construct* the image surface of a specific model using measure-

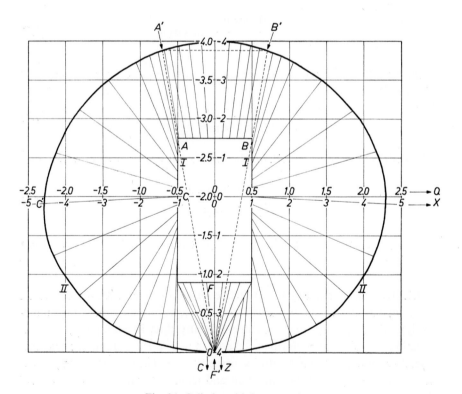

Fig. 34. Cylinder with image surface

ments on the model, we can also, for a simple case, *calculate* it with formulae (if necessary with a digital computer).

7.4.3. We assume a conductive sphere with a (voltage) dipole at the center. The formula given earlier for the potential at distance r from the dipole

$$V = \frac{D_v \cos \theta}{4\pi r^2}$$

which is valid for an infinite space is not adequate for the solution of this problem. There is a boundary condition: no current may pass through the sphere surface: $dV/dn = 0$. This necessitates the addition of an extra term, which furthermore, like the above equation, must satisfy Laplace's law: $\nabla^2 V = 0$. By "trial and error", we find that this term must be $K \cdot r \cdot \cos \theta$ wherein K is a constant which is independent of r and θ, which must be so adapted that it satisfies the boundary condition (it can be shown that $K \cdot r \cdot \cos \theta$ is the only form that satisfies it). If we write

$$V = \frac{D_v \cos \theta}{4\pi r^2} + Kr \cos \theta \qquad (7.6)$$

then, by differentiation of r in $r = a$, we can determine the constant K. The result is:

$$K = \frac{2\,D_v}{4\pi a^3}. \qquad (7.7)$$

The distribution of potential on the sphere surface ($r = a$) now becomes

$$V = \frac{3\,D_v \cos \theta}{4\pi a^2}. \qquad (7.8)$$

Because of symmetry, and also from (7.8) it follows that the image surface is a sphere.

7.4.4. We consider finally a conductive closed cylinder with the dipole on the long axis, above the middle (in fact a crude approximation of the human body). Although with much greater difficulty than in example 3, this calculation can also be performed. (We do not give the computing scheme.) Fig. 34 shows the cylinder with its image surface. The corresponding points are connected by lines, the direction and length of which, as we have said before, *have no significance*.

The lead vector for any pair of electrodes on the actual body can now be directly determined, both in direction and magnitude, by connecting the corresponding points on the image surface.

7.5 General remarks

We can make a few general remarks concerning Figs 33 and 34.

7.5.1. The discontinuities in the direction of the periphery of the body disappear in the image surface, sharp edges being smoothed in the image. Even the image surface is nearly spherical in most cases. A general demonstration of this for the three-dimensional case has not yet been given. It well may be for the two-dimensional case that the image "surface" of a body with any given boundary is a circle. The proof has not yet been published.

7.5.2. If we add "extremities" to the cylinder, they should only be expressed in the image surface as small elevations. This can be understood if we recall that the electric current field penetrates only slightly into the extremities and that thus the difference of potential between two points thereon is small. This must then be expressed in small lead vectors.

7.5.3. It may be asked whether we must limit ourselves to the image *surface* only, or have points *inside* or *outside* this surface physical significance? The answer is affirmative and therefore it is meaningful to speak of an image *space*. We shall explain this.

a. Given that we arrange an electrode inside the body (a method often used today) and that we measure the difference of potential between this and an electrode on the surface. This voltage will be greater, the nearer the internal electrode is to the heart (i.e., the electric source). This appears directly from a consideration of the formula for the potential developed by a dipole (see (6.6), page 39). This implies in the equation (see page 34)

$$V = aX + bY + cZ \tag{6.1}$$

larger values for a, b and c as the inside electrode approaches the heart. Translated into terms of the image space, this will mean that the image point of the internal electrode falls *outside* the image surface (an exact proof of this is lacking). Without going into the background, let it be noted that the image of the heart itself — conceived as a point (dipole) — must be thought of as in infinity.

b. It can be seen that points in the image space *inside* the image surface also have significance. Therefore we assume two electrodes on the body, e.g. R and L. If we connect these via two large resistors r_1 and r_2 with a point S (Fig. 35a) then the difference in potential between any point P and S will be

$$V_S - V_P = \frac{r_1}{r_1 + r_2}(V_L - V_P) + \frac{r_2}{r_1 + r_2}(V_R - V_P). \qquad (7.9)$$

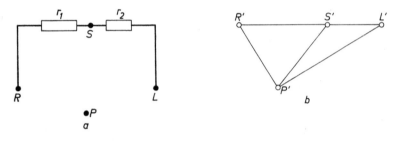

Fig. 35. *a*) By connecting R and L via two resistors we develop point S. *b*) S', the image of S, is on line $R'L'$. It holds $R'S' : S'L' = r_1 : r_2$

If we designate $V_L - V_P \equiv V_1$, $V_R - V_P \equiv V_2$ and $r_1 + r_2 \equiv r_t$, then

$$V_S - V_P = \frac{r_1}{r_t} \cdot V_1 + \frac{r_2}{r_t} \cdot V_2. \qquad (7.10)$$

Applying (6.1) we can write this as

$$V_S - V_P = \left(\frac{a_1 r_1 + a_2 r_2}{r_t}\right)X + \left(\frac{b_1 r_1 + b_2 r_2}{r_t}\right)Y + \left(\frac{c_1 r_1 + c_2 r_2}{r_t}\right)Z$$

$$(7.11)$$

or

$$V_S - V_P = aX + bY + cZ \qquad (7.12)$$

in which a, b and c are the components of the lead vector P at S. It will be readily perceived that S', the image of S, lies on the line connecting R' and L', the said line being divided into segments with the ratio $r_1 : r_2$ (Fig. 35b). S' is inside the image surface.

In general any point can thus be reached inside the image surface by arranging a potentiometer between two electrodes P and Q. The image of the sliding contact is moved by turning the knob, along the connecting line $P' - Q'$.

CHAPTER 8

APPLICATION
OF THE GEOMETRIC REPRESENTATION

In this chapter we shall consider, with reference to a number of examples, how the concept of image space that we have described in the preceding chapter can be applied. Before beginning we must make it clear that we do not make the claim that every application is beneficial in practice or even that the method would be the only one suitable for achieving a specific purpose [1]. On the contrary, a purely analytic approach often performs the required task more exactly and sometimes more rapidly besides. We emphasize the point that analysis is of the first importance. That the concept of the image surface can nonetheless be used with great benefit is shown by what follows:

8.1 Augmented leads

We return again to the Central Terminal (CT) introduced by Wilson (see page 12). The three vertices R', L' and F' which together constitute an oblique triangle (taking the place of Einthoven's equilateral triangle, see page 45) are the image points of the electrode positions on the right arm (R), left arm (L) and left leg (F). We observed that the sides of the triangle have become significant through the introduction of the concept of the lead vector (page 44).

It is now easy to see (page 52 and (3.4), page 13) that the image of the CT is determined at the centre of gravity of the triangle (see Fig. 36a). Naturally also the foot points of the medians can be physically realized. To that end the extremities are connected by large and like resistances to points A, B and C (Fig. 36b). The images of those points, A', B' and C' are determined by transformation and then found to be the middles of the sides of the triangle in the image space (see Fig. 36). (In practice this "distribution" takes place in the apparatus after one or more amplifier stages.)

Instead of the frequently used leads R-CT, L-CT and F-CT, the differences of potential $V_R - V_B$, $V_L - V_C$ and $V_F - V_A$ can now be recorded. Thus results are obtained which are 1.5 times larger than the originals (justifiably designated "*augmented leads*"). This follows geometrically from the fact that

---

[1] Of course: the image space is a geometric representation of analytic data. It never yields more information than does the basis on which it stands.

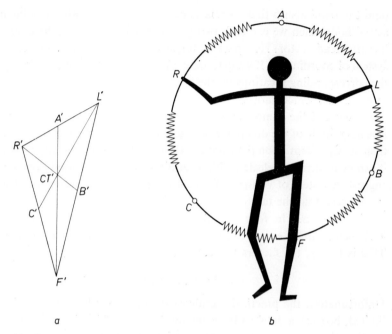

Fig. 36. The foot points of the medians of the lead triangle (*a*) can be realized physically (*b*).

the gravity point of a triangle is met on 1/3 of each of the medians. Algebraically the problem is hardly more complex and anyhow it is a more direct approach. How far the followed reasoning is useful, we leave to the reader's judgement.

8.2 Cubic systems

It would be methodologically advantageous if we could place three pairs of electrodes in such a way that their differences of potential exclusively would be caused by the *x*-, *y*- and *z*-components of the heart vector respectively, hence being proportional to them:

$$X = \alpha_1 V_1, \ Y = \beta_2 V_2, \ Z = \gamma_3 V_3 \tag{8.1}$$

(see (6.4) page 35).

Neither the internal nor the external structure of the human body permit us to rely on natural geometry. But if we know the image surface of the body (and the relationship that correlates each point thereof with a point in the actual body) then we can seek two points thereon, of which the connecting line (the lead vector) runs parallel for instance, to the x-axis of our chosen system of coordinates. If we determine by transformation of these two points the corresponding locations on the human body, we have then found a pair of electrodes which satisfies the said requirement for the x-component.

For each of the components, ∞^2 pairs of points can thus be determined. The magnitude of the difference of potential which can be measured between them is dependent upon the length of the corresponding lead vector and thus it can be arbitrarily selected within certain limits. The method sketched here suggests a system of vectorcardiography containing six electrodes. It will be readily seen that the task can be accomplished with four also, in which case one is common. The four electrodes can even be so selected that the three lead vectors are of equal length (for there are only two degrees of freedom). That is to say, the factors from (8.1) are equal

$$\alpha_1 = \beta_2 = \gamma_3.$$

Unfortunately, the practical usefulness of the matter here discussed is very limited, because a detailed investigation is required for determination of the relationship between image surface and human body.

In conclusion we will observe that the search for the long connecting lines in the image space will lead to determination of electrode locations that yield big differences in potential.

In general we can say that the concept of image space can help us in finding a physically well founded *system of vectorcardiography* (see definition Chapter 9).

CHAPTER 9

TESTING THE DIPOLE APPROXIMATION

By a system of vectorcardiography we understand *a specific choice of electrode locations and a rule for the processing of the measured voltages (the formation of linear combinations) so that in this way three time functions are obtained which — respectively — represent the three components of the heart vector*. If all investigators could agree on one such a system, all other systems now in use (which are often based on intuition) should be discarded in favour of it. With this the uniformity so devoutly wished for and so necessary would be brought into vectorcardiographic research which is an important method additional to electrocardiography and which is being applied in many parts of the world. However obvious this may seem, we can form an idea of what all this really signifies by reflecting that an enormous store of information has been collected in the course of many years — with intuitive systems too. Many cardiologists establish their diagnosis on the basis of their own observations obtained with their own systems. It will therefore certainly not be easy to achieve the ideal referred to above. What steps could be undertaken to draw together the conflicting viewpoints will be discussed elsewhere (Chapter 11).

If a proposal is presented, then of course it is important that the physical basis, hence the representation of the electric activity of the heart by a vector — i.e. the dipole approximation (page 33) — be no longer the subject of doubt. We shall now consider what methods there are to test the accuracy of the dipole approximation, and the conclusion these tests have lead to.

9.1 Cancellation method

Following the historic development, let us first examine a method based on the geometric representation.

We assume the image surface of the human body to be approximately spherical (Fig. 37). (For the sake of clarity an exact sphere is drawn in Fig. 37. No use is made of the properties thereof in the following discussion.) Somewhere on the said surface there lie points R', L' and F'; inside the sphere, at the center of gravity of triangle $R'L'F'$, we find the CT image (Chapter 8, page 54). If we choose an arbitrary point P' on the sphere surface, we can then record the voltage characteristic as a function of time

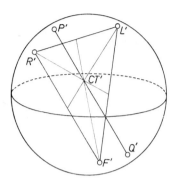

Fig. 37. The image of the human body, represented as a sphere, with images of R, L, F and CT and of two electrodes P and Q, which are antipodal to each other.

between this point and the CT'. (In fact we mean the difference of potential between the electrodes placed at the corresponding points, P on the body and the Central Terminal, determined by transformation. Since hardly any confusion can arise about this, for the sake of the simplicity of our narrative we shall omit this addition in the following pages.)

P will be positive with respect to CT when the projection of the heart vector on line $P'CT'$ "points" at P' and negative, in case this projection points at CT'.

We now put the case that, if the dipole (thus vector) approximation is accurate, there must exist a point Q' such that the difference of potential between Q and CT as a function of time produces a *proportional* curve of *opposite sign* (Fig. 38). This point will of course be the point of intersection of the connecting line $P'CT'$ with the other edge of the sphere (Fig. 39).

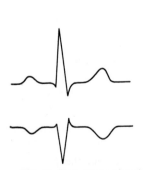

Fig. 38. Two proportional electrocardiograms of opposite sign

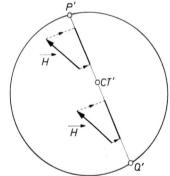

Fig. 39. The projections of H on the lead vectors $P'CT'$ and Q' CT' are equal but the lead vectors are unequal in length.

This can be understood by realising that the projection of the heart vector (H) on $Q'CT'$ will have the same value as the projection on $P'CT'$ but since the lead vector $Q'CT'$ points to the opposite direction in comparison with the lead vector $P'CT'$ the voltage will have the opposite sign.

We can test this in practice by connecting the two leads $V_P - V_{CT}$ and $V_Q - V_{CT}$, furnished with a proportioning factor (a potentiometer), to the same pair of plates of an oscilloscope but in opposition to each other. If a location P is selected anywhere on the body we can try to move electrode Q until, by trial and error, a point is found at which the dot on the screen becomes stationary: the two electrocardiograms exactly balance each other ("*cancellation*").

Control must always be applied in this test by means of the potentiometer, to make the movement of the dot minimal, for $V_Q - V_{CT}$ will only be *proportional* with respect to $V_P - V_{CT}$ and not alike in absolue value, since the lead vectors are generally not equal in lenght (see (7.1) page 41).

That point Q is to be sought experimentally is a consequence of the fact that the image surface of the test individual is not actually known and thus it is impossible to determine Q by transformation from there to the actual surface.

The above described method has a shortcoming, namely that as long as the dot moves on the screen it cannot be seen directly whether this is because the exact point of Q has not been found or whether it is only because the potentiometer is poorly adjusted. Experimentally it is therefore more convenient to use both pairs of oscilloscope plates, connecting a lead to each of them. As long as the exact location of Q has not been determined, a loop appears on the screen that "snaps into" a line when the point sought for is found. Using the potentiometer, it is possible to turn this line until orientation is 45°, at which moment the conditions for the halting of the dot in the first case are established.

A practical difficulty is that by displacing an electrode the measuring apparatus is subjected to such a strong noise signal that the instrument needs some time to recover from the "shock" even when a high speed starter is built into it. This phenomenon makes the experiment combersome and time-consuming, in contrast to the method described below (Chapter 9.2 page 62).

In general, satisfactory results are obtained by the above experiments. It appears to be possible in a great many cases, with a given point P, to find its antipode Q (otherwise, one should be careful in drawing conclusions. See comment, page 65).

However it appears now and then that, even in approximation, one ECG cannot be made successfully to compensate another. This failure of cancellation has also led to the performance of quite different and completely independent experiments. Without going deeply into this we will say a few words about it.

The failure of the cancellation sometimes coincides with a strikingly poor agreement of different systems of vectorcardiography (see Chapter 11). In seeking an explanation of these phenomena we have the choice of two possibilities.

a. The heart itself is the cause. E.g., the dimensions of it could be so great that poles of higher order (see Chapter 14) could play a relatively important role.

b. There is some peculiarity in the conductivity of the tissues outside the heart. To gain more information on this, we should have available heart beats of which the electrical phenomena are completely different from the normal. For these heart beats peculiarities in conductivity *outside* the heart must appear in the same way as they do for normal beats.

Nature itself provides opportunities for experiments of this kind, since atypical heart beats as mentioned above are found in the so-called extrasystoles. For extrasystoles it is true that excitation of the heart is not, in the majority of cases, initiated by the sinu-atrial node, but the heart beat may begin anywhere in the myocardium to spread in a completely abnormal manner over the heart, thereby giving rise to a vectorcardiogram that differs drastically from the normal.

Results of experiments with these extrasystoles appear to have shown that the difficulties must probably be sought not outside but in the heart or on its surface.

Returning to the cancellation, the following should be noted. If in the cases in which compensation is satisfactory, electrode P at the identical location is chosen in various test persons, point Q will by no means be in the identical location. Clearly, individual differences are important. This means that the relationship between the electrocardiogram that can be recorded on the exterior of a human body and the actual electrical phenomena in the heart vary from person to person. It is obvious that as a result of this, essential difficulties arise for the electrocardiography as well as for the vectorcardiography. We will return to these problems later (Chapter 11).

9.2 Becking's method of cancellation

Earlier (page 35) we saw how three arbitrary independent leads can give

us the components of the heart vector (see (6.4)). If we add a fourth lead
to these three (possibly by means of a whole new set of two electrodes) we
can, by analogy with Eq. (6.3) (page 35) write four equations:

$$V_1 = a_1X + b_1Y + c_1Z$$
$$V_2 = a_2X + b_2Y + c_2Z$$
$$V_3 = a_3X + b_3Y + c_3Z \qquad (9.1)$$
$$V_4 = a_4X + b_4Y + c_4Z.$$

If our assumption about the heart vector (that is, the dipole approximation)
is accurate, these four equations are *dependent*. We can then eliminate X,
Y and Z and we obtain:

$$\begin{vmatrix} V_1 & a_1 & b_1 & c_1 \\ V_2 & a_2 & b_2 & c_2 \\ V_3 & a_3 & b_3 & c_3 \\ V_4 & a_4 & b_4 & c_4 \end{vmatrix} = 0.$$

$$(9.2)$$
$$\text{(Becking's equation)}$$

This implies that each of the four differences of potential, independent of
time, can be represented by a linear combination of the three others, e.g.

$$V_4 = p_1V_1 + p_2V_2 + p_3V_3. \qquad (9.3)$$

p_i $(i = 1, 2, 3)$ is the subdeterminant of V_i divided by the subdeterminant
of V_4.

   In this way we have achieved the possibility of performing experiments
similar to those described previously — a kind of generalized cancellation.
For example let V_4 cause the vertical deflection on the oscilloscope screen
while a linear combination of V_1, V_2 and V_3 (to be effected by a balanced
amplifier, potentiometers and switches, in order to be able to adjust the
magnitude and sign of factors p) will be connected to the other pair of plates.
It must now again be possible to let the dot describe a closed line at a 45°
angle (Fig. 40).

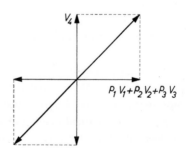

Fig. 40. Becking's method of cancellation

An advantage of this method over the other — as already indicated (page 59) — is that here no electrodes need be displaced, so that the measuring apparatus does not get out of order.

The results are acceptable as in the above discussed cancellation method. That is to say, within a variation of a few percent the goal can be realized. But here also we encounter cases in which the cancellation will not succeed even approximately. As in the first case, we must come to the conclusion that within fairly wide limits vector representation in general yields a good description of the phenomena that we are investigating, but that a more exact examination is needed.

The Becking equation affords not only the possibility of testing dipole approximation. *It also puts us in the position to determine the image surface of a test person.* We shall discuss this in more detail. If we substitute Eq. (9.1) for V_1, V_2, V_3, V_4 in Eq. (9.3) we see immediately that

$$\begin{aligned}
p_1 a_1 + p_2 a_2 + p_3 a_3 &= a_4 \\
p_1 b_1 + p_2 b_2 + p_3 b_3 &= b_4 \\
p_1 c_1 + p_2 c_2 + p_3 c_3 &= c_4
\end{aligned} \qquad (9.4)$$

must be valid. If, in other words, e.g. by *model* measurements, the coordinates (with reference to an arbitrary zero point) of electrodes *1, 2* and *3* are determined in the image space, then it is possible to go further and determine the location on the image surface of any electrode location on the living body (naturally valid only *if* the dipole approximation is valid).

This can be formulated in still another way. We write (9.4) in geometric form:

$$(a_4 b_4 c_4) = p_1 (a_1 b_1 c_1) + p_2 (a_2 b_2 c_2) + p_3 (a_3 b_3 c_3). \qquad (9.5)$$

Factors p_i are scalars. If we assume for the sake of convenience that the four lead vectors $(a_i b_i c_i)$ $(i = 1, 2, 3, 4)$ have the same origin (this means that the four leads $V_i(t)$ have a common electrode) then the lead vector $(a_4 b_4 c_4)$ and hence the location of the fourth unshared electrode can be found in the image space by geometrical means (Fig. 41) after p_1, p_2 and p_3 have been experimentally determined.

One final comment which is analogous to that in Section 9.1: with Eq. (9.4) and Eq. (9.5) we have gained a test of the practical utility of vector representation. For different test individuals we must find like factors p_1, p_2 and p_3 by identical placing of electrodes 1, 2, 3 and 4 and thus the image of electrode 4 must always be found in the same place. In other words, the

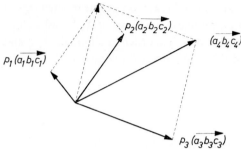

Fig. 41. Geometric (image spatial) representation of Eq. (9.5)

image surface must have the same form and measurements for all subjects. Unfortunately the results of these experiments leave much to be desired, as a result of individual variations. However, the range of discrepancy is such that physically based and practically feasible systems of vectorcardiography can be found.

9.3 Transformation method

Let us assume that we have two systems of vectorcardiography (see Chapter 9 page 57), K and L, such that only three leads play a role in each case (in principle 3 — independent — leads are just enough for determination of the three components of the heart vector, as we have already mentioned several times). These two systems can be defined by three equations each (see (6.4) page 35).

$$
\begin{aligned}
X_K &= \alpha_{1K}V_{1K} + \alpha_{2K}V_{2K} + \alpha_{3K}V_{3K} \\
Y_K &= \beta_{1K}V_{1K} + \beta_{2K}V_{2K} + \beta_{3K}V_{3K} \\
Z_K &= \gamma_{1K}V_{1K} + \gamma_{2K}V_{2K} + \gamma_{3K}V_{3K}
\end{aligned}
\tag{9.6}
$$

and

$$
\begin{aligned}
X_L &= \alpha_{1L}V_{1L} + \alpha_{2L}V_{2L} + \alpha_{3L}V_{3L} \\
Y_L &= \beta_{1L}V_{1L} + \beta_{2L}V_{2L} + \beta_{3L}V_{3L} \\
Z_L &= \gamma_{1L}V_{1L} + \gamma_{2L}V_{2L} + \gamma_{3L}V_{3L}
\end{aligned}
\tag{9.7}
$$

If we realize that neither (X_K, Y_K, Z_K) nor (X_L, Y_L, Z_L) is the actual heart vector but only an approximation, as close as the originator of the system in question could make it, and if we realize also that each of the differences of potential $V_{1K} \ldots V_{3L}$ is a linear function of the true components X,Y,Z of the heart vector then we can understand that the components X_K, Y_K

and Z_K can be written as linear functions of X_L, Y_L and Z_L. For, if $V_{1K} \ldots V_{3L}$ are linear functions of X, Y and Z, we can introduce these functions in (9.6) and (9.7) in order to eliminate X, Y and Z. In general notation the result of this mathematical operation is:

$$
\begin{aligned}
X_K &= P_x X_L + q_x Y_L + r_x Z_L \\
Y_K &= p_y X_L + q_y Y_L + r_y Z_L \\
Z_K &= p_z X_L + q_z Y_L + r_z Z_L.
\end{aligned}
\tag{9.8}
$$

It is obvious that the above statement is only accurate if the dipole approximation is valid. In other words, the testing of the validity of a *linear transformation* of the form of (9.8) — actually (9.8) is none other than a transformation formula — is equivalent to the testing of the dipole approximation.

Anticipating a problem, which we shall discuss in more detail later, we note here that *if* systems K and L should both yield the *same* results, it is valid to say

$$
X_K = X_L \qquad Y_K = Y_L \qquad Z_K = Z_L.
\tag{9.9}
$$

This means that transformation (9.8) is an identical transformation, written as

$$
\begin{pmatrix} p_x & \cdots\cdots & r_x \\ \vdots & & \\ \vdots & & \\ \vdots & & \\ \vdots & & \\ p_z & & r_z \end{pmatrix}
\begin{matrix} 1 \to 1 \\ \\ \end{matrix}
=
\begin{pmatrix} 1 & 0 & 0 \\ 0 & 1 & 0 \\ 0 & 0 & 1 \end{pmatrix}
\tag{9.10}
$$

This actually holds in that when the matrix elements outside the main diagonal are small and the diagonal elements are approximately one, the systems presumably correspond. Both would then in general acceptably approximate the behaviour of the heart vector.

Of course it is possible to verify experimentally the existence of the linear transformation (9.8) by comparing two vectorcardiograms — representatives of systems K and L — taken from the same heart under identical circumstances.

We shall elucidate this with reference to Fig. 42 wherein two "loops" (which must here be thought of as three-dimensional) are drawn. By introduction of time markers into the recording we can seek synchronous (iso-

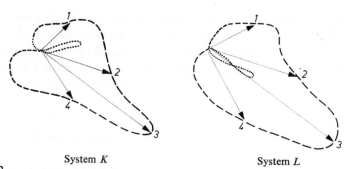

System K System L

Fig. 42.
Two VCG's, representatives of two systems of vectorcardiography. The arrows indicate
the heart vector in isophasal positions.

phasal) points and measure the coordinates X_{iK}, Y_{iK} ... Z_{iL}. For each pair
of points K, L equation (9.8) must be satisfied. The nine coefficients p_x ... r_z
are not known, however. We can find them by considering three pairs of
points ($i = 1, 2, 3$) with which $3 \times 3 = 9$ equations can be set up so that they
can be solved for the nine coefficients. If we now select an arbitrary fourth
pair of points and substitute their coordinates in the system of three equations according to (9.8) with the coefficients calculated for them, we will
encounter no contradictions, on condition ..... that the dipole approximation is valid!

Naturally the values of p_x ... r_z are not completely independent from the
selection of points i. For that reason in practice preferably more than three
are selected so that for the said nine unknowns more equations exist. Using
the method of least squares — and an electronic computer — we obtain
values that are as closely as possible representative for the case in question.

The results of these experiments are about the same as to the preceding
tests, that is that rather fitting linear transformations are found, especially
for one and the same individual. However, by comparing coefficients
p_x ... r_z, computed for various test persons (and, of course, using only the
systems K and L) it appears that there is some divergence which makes clear
that the relationship between systems K and L is not the same for every one.

9.4 Conclusions

We will make one more comment before we come to our final conclusion.
We consider two entirely independent "loops", not too capricious, but apart

from that fully *arbitrarily* drawn. It appears that a linear relationship can almost always be found and that one figure can be transformed with reasonable accuracy into the other (this is not true of very detailed figures). It can happen that this phenomenon is in force here, so that a transformation that tallies is no guarantee of the validity of the dipole approximation. This is in contrast with the transformation that does not tally — as may primarily be the case with winding loops — in which the approximation must naturally be rejected directly. We must therefore handle our results meticulously.

Our final conclusion, by analogy with the earlier one is this: the dipole approximation for every test individual certainly does not in itself deserve to be discarded and it can doubtless serve as a reasonable provisional working base, but the individual differences are of such a nature that an adaptation and extension of theory and method deserve full consideration (see Chapter 14).

CHAPTER 10

THE TOTAL DIPOLE AND CORRECTED SYSTEMS

10.1 General

Up to this point in our discussion we have always proceeded from the dipole approximation, i.e.: the electrical heart activity can be represented by a vector, the dipole moment belonging to a dipole which is stationary with respect to place. In the preceding chapters we have seen that this representation can lead in general to satisfactory results, but that sometimes the approximation fails. It is therefore reasonable to extend our hypothesis. We do this by assuming a *collection of dipoles* and by investigating to what extent the distribution of potential on the body *surface* yields information on distribution of dipole density *in* the body.

This idea can be rejected immediately in such a formulation because fundamentally *it is not possible to determine the dipole distribution in a body by measurement of the potential distribution at the surface* (a conclusion already reached by Gauss with reference to the matter of the origin of terrestrial magnetism).

The uncertainty of this problem will be demonstrated by a simple example: we imagine a closed surface with a homogeneous distribution of voltage dipoles thereon. Then to each surface element we can ascribe a dipole moment, perpendicular and in size proportional to the area of the element (Fig. 43). It can be established that such a closed dipole layer has a dis-

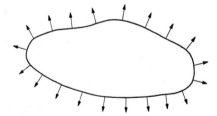

Fig. 43. Homogeneous closed dipole layer

continuity of the electric field at the layer. This potential jump will be equal anywhere at the surface. As a result of it an arbitrary potential distribution somewhere outside the closed surface, will not be influenced by the presence of this surface, no matter what the configuration thereof. It is relevant to our problem that if one or more homogeneous closed dipole layers are to be added to a specific dipole distribution in the heart, the potential distribution on the body surface must not be altered. Conversely, a given potential distribution on the body surface yields no decisive information on the internal dipole distribution. What can be determined from the potential distribution, however, is *the total dipole effect*, hence the total dipole moment, of any dipole distribution within a body, whereas the body is a homogeneous and isotropic medium. The theoretical solution of the problem a few years ago (1954) by Gabor and Nelson was — like the result — astonishingly simple.

10.2 Theory of Gabor and Nelson

A space (Fig. 44) is assumed, insulated from the exterior and consisting, as already noted, of a homogeneous and isotropic medium. In the space

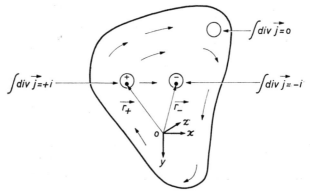

Fig. 44. Positive and negative current poles in an insulated homogeneous and isotropic medium

the authors posit a collection of positive and negative current poles, so that the current field **j** in the body comprises as a *totality* neither positive nor negative sources, hence:

$$\int_{\text{vol}} \text{div } \boldsymbol{j} \, dv = 0. \tag{10.1}$$

We can formulate the insulated condition of the body by noting that the normal component of the current density at the boundary is zero. In other words,

$$\boldsymbol{j} \perp d\boldsymbol{S}. \tag{10.2}$$

We now consider one positive and one negative pole which deliver a current i passing into and out of the body respectively. The radius vectors at these poles from the source of an arbitrarily assumed system of coordinates are designated r_+ and r_-. The product of current intensity i and the vector $(r_+ - r_-)$ is designated D_i, the "doublet strength":

$$D_i = i(r_+ - r_-) \tag{10.3}$$

(as we indicated earlier (page 29), in the limits $(r_+ - r_-) \to 0$ and $i \to \infty$, D_i is the dipole moment). We shall see how this expression (10.3) can be generalized. We begin with a step which is perhaps not entirely justifiable mathematically, but which none the less leads to a satisfactory result. We imagine each pole to be "spread-out" over a volume element Δv. It will be immediately seen that the divergence of the current density, integrated over the volume element, yields the current i that passes at the pole. Thus, for a positive pole

$$\int_{\Delta v} \operatorname{div} j \, dv = i \tag{10.4a}$$

(wherein $\Delta v \gg dv$) and, by analogy, for a negative pole

$$\int_{\Delta v} \operatorname{div} j \, dv = -i. \tag{10.4b}$$

This is all valid for any current doublet in the body. Naturally everywhere where there are no poles

$$\int_{\Delta v} \operatorname{div} j \, dv = 0. \tag{10.4c}$$

Without going into the problems of singularities, we assume that (10.4a) and (10.4b) will be valid when we proceed from current *doublets* to current *dipoles*. It is then clear that for the total dipole moment, caused by an arbitrary collection of current dipoles, we can write

$$D_i = \int_{\text{vol}} r \operatorname{div} j \, dv. \tag{10.5}$$

We shall demonstrate that this expression can be associated with the potential distribution, as we are able to measure it on the body surface.

We first consider the x-component of (10.5):

$$(D_i)_x = \int_{\text{vol}} x \operatorname{div} j \, dv. \tag{10.6}$$

According to a rule of vector calculation

$$\text{div } (x\boldsymbol{j}) = x \text{ div } \boldsymbol{j} - \boldsymbol{j} \cdot \text{grad } x \qquad (10.7)$$

so that

$$(D_i)_x = \int_{\text{vol}} \text{div } (x\boldsymbol{j}) dv - \int_{\text{vol}} \boldsymbol{j} \cdot \text{grad } x \ dv. \qquad (10.8)$$

According to Gauss' theorem we can write the first term as

$$\int_{\text{vol}} \text{div } (x\boldsymbol{j}) dv = \int_{\text{surface}} x\boldsymbol{j} \ d\boldsymbol{S} = 0 \qquad (10.9)$$

for $\boldsymbol{j} \perp d\boldsymbol{S}$ (see 10.2). Thus

$$(D_i)_x = - \int_{\text{vol}} \boldsymbol{j} \cdot \text{grad } x \ dv = - \int_{\text{vol}} j_x \ dv. \qquad (10.10)$$

We saw earlier that $\boldsymbol{j} = -\sigma \boldsymbol{\nabla} V$ (Equation (5.13) page 28) whereby we get

$$(D_i)_x = \sigma \iiint \frac{\partial V}{\partial x} dx \ dy \ dz. \qquad (10.11)$$

Integrating according to x gives

$$(D_i)_x = \sigma \iint V \ dy \ dz \qquad (10.12)$$

wherein $V = V_1 - V_2$ (see Fig. 45) (V_2 in the negative x-direction, is here assumed to be negative), $dy \ dz$ is the x-component of surface element $d\boldsymbol{S}$. Thus

$$(D_i)_x = \sigma \int_{\text{surface}} V(d\boldsymbol{S})_x. \qquad (10.13a)$$

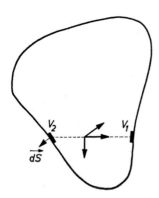

Fig. 45. $V = V_1 - V_2$ (see (10.12))

Analogous treatment of y- and z-components of $\boldsymbol{D}_i$ yields

$$(D_i)_y = \sigma \int_{\text{surface}} V(dS)_y \qquad (10.13b)$$

$$(D_i)_z = \sigma \int_{\text{surface}} V(dS)_z. \qquad (10.13c)$$

If we now combine the components, we obtain

$$\boldsymbol{D}_i = \sigma \int_{\text{surface}} V \, d\boldsymbol{S} \qquad (10.14)$$

This expression is indeed astonishingly simple: To obtain the total dipole moment it is merely necessary to integrate the potential [1]) over the entire body surface, *whereby the question of the point of application of the heart vector — thus the fixedness of the dipole — is eliminated.*

10.3 Verification of the theory

Before we go into the practical significance of (10.14) we will demonstrate the result in yet another fashion, because this equation has had such an important effect on the further development of vectorcardiography. We are starting from an expression that was used earlier

$$j = \sigma(-\boldsymbol{\nabla} V + \boldsymbol{E}^*) \qquad (5.11)$$

(see pages 27 and 30) where $\boldsymbol{E}^*$ is the so-called electromotive field strength, the origin of the electric activity of the heart.

We consider, as before, a homogeneous conductive and infinite space. In a spherical volume separated from this space we imagine a homogeneous electromotive field strength $\boldsymbol{E}^*$ caused by diffusion and membrane effect. As deduced in Chapter 5, for the potential at a point anywhere outside the sphere, we can write (in polar coordinates r and θ) (see page 32)

$$V = \frac{E^* \cos \theta \cdot \text{volume sphere}}{4\pi r^2}. \qquad (5.23)$$

---

[1]) It seems contradictory to what has been said earlier, to speak here of *"the potential"* and not *potential differences.* It is not a contradiction however, because nothing is changed when we sum a constant at V. Integrated over the whole closed surface this constant makes no contribution.

For an arbitrary volume that can be thought of as built up from a collection of globules of various magnitudes, this expression goes over into an integral (see (5.24) page 32)

$$V = \frac{\int\limits_{\text{vol}} E^* \cos\theta \, dv}{4\pi r^2}.$$ (10.15)

We can also think of this potential as originating from a current dipole placed in the origin of the system of coordinates. Here also we deduced an expression (see page 29).

$$V = \frac{D_i \cos\theta}{4\pi\sigma r^2}.$$ (5.17)

We can identify D_i here, obviously, with the total dipole. By making (10.15) and (5.17) equal we obtain

$$D_i = \sigma \int E^* \, dv.$$ (10.16)

If we substitute (5.11) in this expression, we obtain

$$D_i = \sigma \int \nabla V \, dv + \int j \, dv.$$ (10.17)

The second term of the right-hand member will be scrutinized more closely. In agreement with Gabor and Nelson, we assume that in the volume in question there is neither positive nor negative source, and hence that div $j = 0$. This implies that the lines along which the electricity moves must be closed. Let us consider one of the flow tubes and perform the integration $\int j \, dv$. We see (Fig. 46) that the volume dv of a length of the tube along dl can be written as $dv = dS \, dl$, because dS is the surface of the cross section. If we consider that vector j is always directed along the line of flow, then

$$\int j \, dv = \int j \, dS \, dl.$$ (10.18)

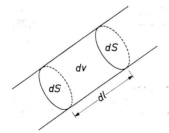

Fig. 46. A flow tube with cross section dS

Here $j\,dS$ is the amount of electricity that flows through the tube per unit of time, hence, the current intensity. This magnitude, since div $j = 0$, is constant so that

$$\int j\, dS\, dl = j\, dS \int dl. \qquad (10.19)$$

The last integral is zero, because the lines of current flow are closed, as noted above. Thus

$$\int j\, dv = 0. \qquad (10.20)$$

We now rewrite the first term, by analogy with what we determined in the first calculation

$$\sigma \int_{\text{vol}} \boldsymbol{\nabla} V\, dv = \sigma \int_{\text{surface}} V\, dS \qquad (10.21)$$

(Gauss) (equations (10.11) and (10.13a)) so that finally we obtain

$$\boldsymbol{D_i} = \sigma \int_{\text{surface}} V\, dS \qquad (10.14)$$

the same result as that of Gabor and Nelson (see page 71).

What are the consequences of the above calculations for the practice of vectorcardiography? It is true that the result seems very attractive, but strictly speaking we have hardly made any progress because in these deductions our point of departure has always been a homogeneous body, while a man is not at all homogeneous. It is possible to think up various arguments for leaving out of consideration this human lack of homogeneity. This implies however that only an "effective dipole" can be sought, which we must assume to be present somewhere in the body, and that must be such that the phenomena on the surface of the body must correspond to it as closely as possible (see page 37). If we do this, we may apply the formulae above. It is obvious that *in practice we are not able actually to determine an integral. We must therefore be content with the construction of a sum* that more closely approximates actuality as the number of terms increases.

We shall now review some systems of vectorcardiography which attempt to realize the goal in various ways, and which all have the common characteristic that they use more electrodes than the minimum of four [1]) which was

---

[1]) i.e., three independent leads.

necessary according to the previously discussed dipole approximation, for determination of the three components of the heart vector.

10.4 The BW-system (Burger)

First we discuss an attempt to combine two systems mentioned above. One system consists of three limb electrodes: right arm (R), left arm (L) and left leg (F) and a fourth electrode (W) on the back according to Wilson's system (see page 20). The second system also makes use of the extremities, but the fourth electrode is on the chest (B). For the sake of convenience we designate the respective systems RLFW and RLFB.

If we consider these possibilities separately, we can anticipate flaws in each. To assess the significance of these flaws we recall that the heart is anteriorly placed in the thorax and that its dimensions are not negligible with respect to those of the thorax. This means that part of the electrical activity that is caused by the anterior part of the heart influences electrode B more (i.e. it will impart to B a greater difference in potential with respect to the other electrodes) than a similar activity generated by the posterior part of the heart. The reverse will naturally be the case with the electrode on the back, though to a lesser degree because the relative difference of distance between the front and back of the heart and W is less.

We can attempt to mitigate this drawback, which is a result of the finite dimension of the heart (better, the great spread of the dipole plane, see Chapters 14 and 15) by combining both systems and thereby providing each with one or another weight factor as expressed below

$$\alpha(RLFW) + \beta(RLFB) \tag{10.22}$$

whereby

$$\alpha + \beta = 1 \tag{10.23}$$

A possible choice is $\alpha = 1/3$, $\beta = 2/3$. In this connection it must be noted that the relationship between α and β is not especially critical if $RLFW$ and $RLFB$ are well founded systems, and even that they might be selected with complete arbitrariness if both systems independently would yield identical results. (In that case the dipole approximation must be assumed to be exactly and generally valid and thus combinations in general would be without meaning.)

In practice the procedure has been as follows. In the first place the coefficients of the $RLFW$ system are adapted as closely as possible to those of

RLFB. This is done on the basis of the — not exactly valid — dipole approximation, and by means of the method described in Section 9.2. Briefly reviewed: when the locations of four electrodes (here *R*, *L*, *F* and *B*) are determined in the image space by model measurements, it is possible, applying a cancellation experiment, to determine which linear combination (Equations (9.4) and (9.5)) of the three lead vectors yields the lead vector of the fifth electrode (*W*). Different results (Fig. 47) are obtained for different

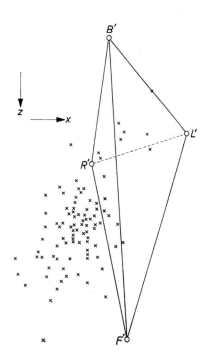

Fig. 47. Measured results from determination of the location of *W'* in the image space

test individuals, and these results are averaged. The resulting electrode positions are shown in Fig. 48. Next we determine to what extent these systems overlap or, better, what differences they exhibit. It appears that the differences in the vectorcardiograms thus produced are not particularly large, but insofar as they are present they afford occasion for a directed but not especially critical choice of α and β. The two systems must now be combined according to the still rather vague formula (10.22). We shall explain it in more detail. In accordance with the dipole approximation we can write a set of three equations for each system, whereby the three components of the

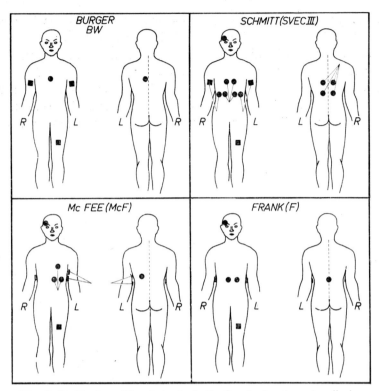

Fig. 48. Positioning of the electrodes in the four lead systems described

heart vector are expressed in the three independent potential differences, e.g. for *RLFW*

$$X_a = a_{11}V_{WR} + a_{12}V_{FR} + a_{13}V_{LR}$$
$$Y_a = a_{21}V_{WR} + a_{22}V_{FR} + a_{23}V_{LR} \qquad (10.24)$$
$$Z_a = a_{31}V_{WR} + a_{32}V_{FR} + a_{33}V_{LR}.$$

Similarly for system *RLFB*

$$X_b = b_{11}V_{BR} + b_{12}V_{FR} + b_{13}V_{LR}$$
$$Y_b = b_{21}V_{BR} + b_{22}V_{FR} + b_{23}V_{LR} \qquad (10.25)$$
$$Z_b = b_{31}V_{BR} + b_{32}V_{FR} + b_{33}V_{LR}.$$

The combination is then written as

$$X = \alpha X_a + \beta X_b$$
$$Y = \alpha Y_a + \beta Y_b \qquad (10.26)$$
$$Z = \alpha Z_a + \beta Z_b.$$

We see from this that each component of the heart vector is no longer determined by three potential differences, but rather by four. With this system
of vectorcardiography an initial attempt is reported, *to become more independent of the position of the total dipole by use of more electrodes than the
minimal four.* We designated this a *"corrected system"*.

10.5 The F-system (Frank)

This one, which is also a "corrected system", uses seven electrodes (see
Fig. 48). Whereas in the *B* system measurements on a model which is *not
homogeneous* are used, in combination with results from experiments with
test individuals, Frank based his work entirely on measurements on a homogeneous model. In this model the location of the dipole, the artificial heart,
is varied while for each case extensive measurements of the potential distribution on the surface are made. From them a system is developed whereby
the electrodes are placed in such a way that the effect of a displacement of
the dipole on the difference of potential between the electrodes is as slight
as possible. Thus each component of the heart vector is formed by a linear
combination of six differences of potential (indicated by Frank in the form
of a system of resistors, as well as by coefficients).

10.6 The S-system (Schmitt)

A method which is not substantially different from that of Frank is given
by Schmitt, who also based his system on measurements on a homogeneous
model. The number of electrodes is expanded here to fourteen (Fig. 48). Some
are combined as a group by means of resistors in such a way that individual
differences of position of the heart and the dipole distribution are averaged
out. Otherwise the way in which the electrodes are located recalls to a certain
extent the old desire to obtain the three components of the heart vector
directly "in the form of a voltage" (we bear in mind the fact that *the unit
of a dipole moment is Vcm²* !). This now occurs, in contrast to earlier systems,
(see page 21) in a way that has a firm physical basis.

10.7 The M-system (McFee)

In this section we shall, as in the first case, treat the basis of the system
rather extensively. McFee used the law of reciprocals, already established in

the last century by Helmholtz. We review the process of this calculation, whereafter the result will be adapted to the problems of vectorcardiography.

We use Green's theorem which for any function φ and ψ reads:

$$\int_{\text{vol}} [\varphi(r)\triangledown^2\psi(r) - \psi(r)\triangledown^2\varphi(r)]dv = \int_{\text{surface}} [\varphi(r)\boldsymbol{\nabla}\psi(r) - \psi(r)\boldsymbol{\nabla}\varphi(r)]dS \qquad (10.27)$$

or, in another notation

$$\int_{\text{vol}} [\varphi(x,y,z)\triangledown^2\psi(x,y,z) - \psi(x,y,z)\triangledown^2\varphi(x,y,z)]dv =$$
$$\int_{\text{surface}} \left[\varphi(x,y,z)\frac{d\psi(x,y,z)}{dn} - \psi(x,y,z)\frac{d\varphi(x,y,z)}{dn}\right]dS \qquad (10.28)$$

in which $\triangledown^2$ is the Laplace operator and n is the normal vector on the closed surface over which integration is to be performed, positive when directing at the outside.

In the following $\varphi(x,y,z)$ and $\psi(x,y,z)$ are potentials.

We consider a closed surface (Fig. 49) within which there is a homogeneous conducting medium. We imagine two point sources, 1 and 2. From these sources there is delivered current i_1 and i_2, provisionally positive and of any magnitude, each leading to a potential field V_1 and V_2. To prevent an accumulation of electric charge, the currents which are introduced must be carried off. We assume that this discharge occurs uniformly over the entire surface. This implies that at the surface $dV/dn \neq 0$; particularly we chose $dV/dn = $ constant for both V_1 and V_2. (How this can be accomplished in actuality is not the question: we use this only as a mathematical artifice.)

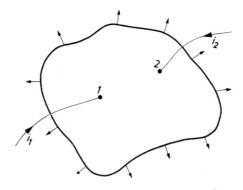

Fig. 49. Two punctate positive current sources in a homogeneous medium

On the superposed potential fields excited by i_1 and i_2 we adapt Green's theorem. According to (10.28)

$$\int_v (V_1 \nabla^2 V_2 - V_2 \nabla^2 V_1)dv = \int_s \left(V_1 \frac{dV_2}{dn} - V_2 \frac{dV_1}{dn} \right)dS \quad (10.29)$$

must then be valid. In the lefthand member

$$\int_v V_1 \nabla^2 V_2 \, dv = 0 \quad (10.30)$$

everywhere except for a volume element (Δv_2) in the immediate vicinity of source 2 (see also Eq. (5.6) and (5.8) page 26). We now introduce the following notation: $(V_1)_2 =$ the potential at point 2, caused by the current flowing into the medium at 1, and similarly for other combinations. We realize that V_1 is practically constant in Δv_2, so that

$$\int_{\Delta v_2} V_1 \nabla^2 V_2 \, dv = (V_1)_2 \int_{\Delta v_2} \nabla^2 V_2 \, dv = -(V_1)_2 \frac{i_2}{\sigma}. \quad (10.31)$$

By substituting Eq. (10.31) we obtain for the left-hand member of Eq. (10.29)

$$\int_v (V_1 \nabla^2 V_2 - V_2 \nabla^2 V_1)dv = -(V_1)_2 \frac{i_2}{\sigma} + (V_2)_1 \frac{i_1}{\sigma}. \quad (10.32)$$

From the right-hand member of (10.29) we consider $\int_s V_1 \, dV_2/dn \cdot dS$. As previously set as a condition, $dV_2/dn =$ constant. Thus this term may be put before the integral. Dividing by — and multiplying with — S then, as readily can be seen we obtain

$$\int_s V_1 \frac{dV_2}{dn} \, dS = \frac{dV_2}{dn} S \frac{\int_s V_1 dS}{S} = -\frac{i_2}{\sigma} \bar{V}_1 \quad (10.33)$$

in which $\bar{V}_1$ is the potential caused by source 1 averaged over the surface. We thus determine the whole right-hand member of Eq. (10.29)

$$\int_s \left(V_1 \frac{dV_2}{dn} - V_2 \frac{dV_1}{dn} \right)dS = -\frac{i_2}{\sigma} \bar{V}_1 + \frac{i_1}{\sigma} \bar{V}_2. \quad (10.34)$$

(10.32) and (10.34) combined yield the equation

$$(V_1)_2 i_2 - (V_2)_1 i_1 = -i_1 \bar{V}_2 + i_2 \bar{V}_1 \tag{10.35}$$

The relationship, as the result of a general example, will be adapted to a more specific case, from which again we are able to adapt to vectorcardiography.

We consider once more a homogeneous conducting body with four current sources, A, B, C and D rather than two. If we introduce a current i_1 at A and carry it off at B while we do the same with i_2 at C and D, we may assume the body to be insulated and thus abandon the rather artificial method of taking off the current over the surface (Fig. 50). We now for a

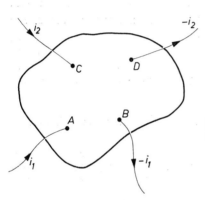

Fig. 50. Two positive and two negative current sources in the homogeneous medium

moment consider only points A and C (because at these points only current can be introduced into the body we still have to make use of the assumption $dV/dn = $ constant). In accordance with (10.35) we can write

$$(V_C)_A i_1 - (V_A)_C i_2 = i_1 \bar{V}_C - i_2 \bar{V}_A. \tag{10.36}$$

A similar expression is valid for points B and C, in that manner that for the current at point B the value $-i_1$ must be assigned:

$$(V_C)_B i_1 - (V_B)_C i_2 = -i_1 \bar{V}_C - i_2 \bar{V}_B. \tag{10.37}$$

If we add (10.36) and (10.37), then

$$(V_C)_{AB} i_1 - (V_{AB})_C i_2 = -i_2(\bar{V}_A + \bar{V}_B) \tag{10.38}$$

in which $(V_C)_{AB}$ represents the difference of potential between points A and B, caused by i_2 in C, while $(V_{AB})_C$ is the potential at C, the result of i_1 and $-i_1$. (Since the conducting wires can carry off the charge, we can replace the artificial dV/dn = constant with $dV/dn = 0$.)

It can readily be seen that a similar formulation appears when instead of C the point D is taken (whereby, as previously, we substitute $-i_2$ for i_2) thus

$$(V_D)_{AB}i_1 + (V_{AB})_D i_2 = i_2(\bar{V}_A + \bar{V}_B) \tag{10.39}$$

We can now add (10.38) and (10.39) with the result

$$(V_{CD})_{AB}i_1 = (V_{AB})_{CD}i_2 \tag{10.40}$$

where of course $dV/dn = 0$. This is the principle of reciprocals of Helmholtz, symmetrical at AB and CD.

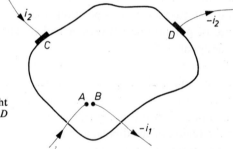

Fig. 51. Points A and B are brought near each other to a dipole. C and D are placed on the surface

Following McFee we shall adapt this result to vectorcardiography. We let points A and B approach until they are so close together that we can speak of a current dipole. At the same time we permit C and D to separate, and especially we select locations for them on the body surface (Fig. 51). We now allow a current to pass from A to B and from C to D and apply the theorem of reciprocals to our case, adapted to the indicated situation. We can express the difference of potential between A and B, $(V_{CD})_{AB}$, as the scalar product of the field strength $(E_{CD})_{AB}$ between A and B, and the vector AB.

For the voltage between C and D we use the same expression that we had before for the difference of potential between two electrodes, caused by a dipole somewhere in the body, namely the scalar product of lead vector abc with dipole moment XYZ (Equation (7.1) page 44), thus

$$(E_{CD})_{AB} \cdot AB \cdot i_1 = abc \cdot XYZ \cdot i_2 \tag{10.41}$$

Since AB is a current dipole and XYZ is a voltage dipole, the second term becomes

$$abc \cdot YXZ \cdot i_2 = abc \cdot \frac{D_1}{\sigma} \cdot i_2 = abc \cdot \frac{AB \cdot i_1}{\sigma} \cdot i_2 \qquad (10.42)$$

(see page 29). Since (10.42) is valid for any AB, Equation (10.41) becomes

$$\sigma(E_{CD})_{AB} = i_2 \cdot abc \qquad (10.43)$$

or

$$(j_{CD})_{AB} = i_2 \cdot abc. \qquad (10.44)$$

This is an important result, for we now see that, aside from one constant factor, the current density and the lead vector are the same. We adapt this to the following example. If we assume that a current i is carried through the human body from the left arm to the right, then the current field at an arbitrary place in the body corresponds with the lead vector for electrodes R and L in case a dipole is positioned in the same place giving rise to a difference of potentional between R and L. The current field in this association is designated "*lead field*".

We may now put the following case. Given two electrodes on the body surface and a dipole placed somewhere inside the body. If we say that the voltage between the electrodes may not be dependent upon the location of the dipole then this statement is equivalent to: the current field (lead field) in the region of the dipole, as a result of a current carried from one electrode to the other, must be homogeneous.

Generalizing for more electrodes: for an ideal lead system a combination of differences of potential between various electrodes should be such that the precise location of the total dipole in the heart has no role. Using the reciprocals theorem we can also state the case thus: a combination of currents, controlled by the various electrodes must deliver a *homogeneous* lead field at the location of the heart.

With this remark we return in fact to the Gabor and Nelson formula (10.14) which in principle presents a method for determining the total dipole moment independent of the location of the dipole.

Experimentally the problem can be attacked this way. Control an electric current by a plurality of electrodes in a model and vary the positions of the electrodes in such a way that at the location of the heart a homogeneous lead field is developed. The electrodes which rationally meet this requirement, will, with the correct coefficients — conversely — be usable for determination of the total dipole moment.

McFee did not work with an electric current, but with a fluid flow which he allowed to pass over granules of $KMnO_4$ in a glass model (originally two-dimensional and heterogeneous, later three-dimensional and homogeneous). The current field here was represented by purple lines.

The result of McFee's experiment was a system of nine electrodes. Fig. 48 page 76 indicates how they are distributed over the body.

In all this we must remind ourselves that in principle it is *impossible* to meet the requirement of a homogeneous lead field at the location of the heart, caused by a current controlled by a plurality of electrodes. Blood, myocardium and other kinds of tissue do not all exhibit the same conductivity. This implies a refraction of the current lines and thus, in transition from one medium to another, there is a bend, therefore excluding homogeneity.

This means that we must assume the effective dipole (i.e. the dipole that produces the field as satisfactorily as possible, measured at the body surface) to be located in a "heart cavity" filled with a homogeneous conducting medium. But what conductivity must we chose? A firm choice is not to be made, and therewith there remains an essential imponderable in the problem.

This does not mean that it would not be desirable to find a medically usable system that is grounded in physics as solidly as possible, but it is well to bear this principal limitation in mind.

In this connection we emphatically warn against the numerous, but inaccurate opinions that are advanced, as though all difficulties and uncertainties concerning relationship between the electric activity of the heart and the leads were specific to vectorcardiography. *Of course these problems are basic to electrocardiography too*, but most users in that field are not conscious about them (see also page 60).

Still one more system must be mentioned, namely that of Rylant. This system uses 72 electrodes which, to meet the requirement of practical usability, are held in a flexible rubber vest so that patients with different body measurements can easily be examined. The electrodes are interconnected by a passive network of resistors. Although the author states the grounds inadequately in his publications, he suggests that in the theoretical background use can be made of the properties of non Euclidian space. As a consequence of the complexity of the problem, it is not yet possible to value this system.

CHAPTER 11

SUBJECTIVE AND OBJECTIVE COMPARISON OF SYSTEMS OF VECTORCARDIOGRAPHY

COMPROMISE IN VECTORCARDIOGRAPHY

In all possibilities for the designs of vectorcardiography systems it is of course of very great importance to establish a criterion whereby it is possible to estimate the extent to which the vectorcardiogram obtained by a given system, actually is representative of electric events in the heart, and also to estimate its practical value. In the preceding chapters it has become evident that the ideal system does not exist. It is not possible to judge a system on its individual merits and we must therefore proceed by no other means than comparison, that is to say, find out to what degree the results of two systems are in agreement.

We shall apply two working methods: *subjective* and *objective*.

11.1 Subjective comparison

This method is very simple in nature and is based on nothing other than the assigning of an evaluation in figures from 0 to 10. The procedure is as follows: Two vectorcardiograms of the same patient, obtained with the two systems under comparison are judged by three experts who express their evaluation concerning correlation by means of a figure. If the evaluations differ only slightly, they are averaged and then rounded off to a whole number. If there is a greater deviation between evaluations than the doubt which the compilers felt in making their judgements, then a consultation is held, to reach a consensus. If this is done for a great number of patients, a reasonable impression is finally obtained as to the degree in which two systems correspond.

The subjective element in this method of comparison lies primarily in the fact that special emphasis will be laid on characteristics that are of diagnostic importance, rather than on purely geometric data. Thus for example in frontal and horizontal projection the proportion of maximum deflection in the x-direction on either side of the center of the loop is important (so-called right-left ratio). Furthermore, for example, the direction of the circulation of the loop is of essential diagnostic significance, whereas on the contrary the size of the loop is of less interest.

If in the comparison of a new series of vectorcardiograms the preceding one is kept in mind, the assessor attains a true continuity in the meaning of the figures.

The result of a comparison (in approximately 175 cases) of the four corrected systems described in the preceding chapter is shown in Fig. 52. Only the frontal and horizontal projections are presented (Fig. 14, page 21 and Fig. 15, page 22). This has its basis in the nature of the instrumentation: at the time of this investigation the vectorcardiograph was not yet developed for recording of the sagittal projection. (The compilers of the present scheme were aware of course that the three components were not evenly evaluated).

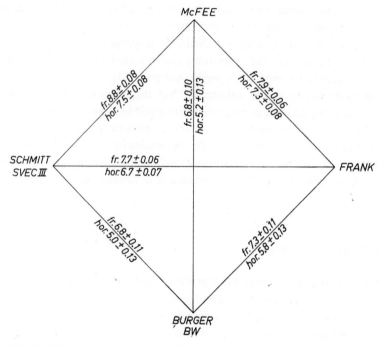

Fig. 52. Diagram showing the subjective comparison of four lead systems

In each evaluation in Fig. 52 the standard error is shown, determined in the customary way by application of the formula

$$\text{standard error} = \sqrt{\left(\dfrac{\sum\limits_{i}\left(x_i - \bar{x}\right)^2}{n(n-1)}\right)}.\tag{11.1}$$

We observe the following in Fig. 52.

a. In the comparison of any pair of systems it appears that the frontal projection significantly is always judged more favorably than the horizontal. This is certainly due to the fact that the sagittal component was so strongly affected by the circumstance that in the z-direction (Fig. 14, page 21) the heart has relatively such large dimensions, as a consequence of which there is a great difference between an excitation at the front and one at the back of the heart. These geometric differences have less significance for the other two components.

b. The mutual correlation between the Schmitt, McFee and Frank systems is clearly better than between Burger's and the other three. The cause of this may be sought inter alia in the corresponding and/or differentiating starting points from which the respective systems are developed. In Utrecht the starting point was distinctly heterogeneous models and test individuals, whereas the other three systems are based on measurements on homogeneous models (however, see page 83).

c. All four systems ignore anisotropy. Yet this phenomenon must play a not insignificant role, as measurements made in the course of years have indicated that the conductivity in the lengthwise direction of muscle is approximately 15 times that which one obtains in the transverse direction. But the way in which the anisotropy might be brought into the calculation is still so obscure that for the present it is disregarded.

11.2 Objective comparison

We indicated earlier (page 64) that if the dipole approximation is accurate, it must always be possible to establish a *linear transformation* which converts two arbitrary systems, each with four or more electrodes, into each other. If we drop the dipole approximation and proceed on the basis of the Gabor-Nelson theory, in systems with four or more independent leads (thus systems "corrected" for the extent and displacement of the dipole layer, see Chapter 14 and 15), then in principle we will no longer anticipate such a linear relationship.

We run into trouble especially when we calculate a transform matrix for one patient and attempt to adapt it to another. Results are better if we try to develop an *average transformation* from a broader material. Such a linear relationship then appears to have a right to existance, as it concerns the omparison of systems averaged over many individuals. It is for this reason

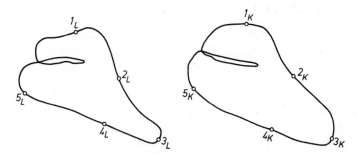

Fig. 53. *a*) VCG from *L* system
b) VCG from *K* system
Only one projection is sketched in this figure

that we shall consider in greater detail the general method that can be used
in seeking this average transformation.

We consider, as in Section 9.3 page 65, two vectorcardiograms (Fig. 53)
representing two systems L and K. On loop L we select one or another point
and then the isophasal point on loop K, and we designate the coordinates X_L,
Y_L, Z_L and X_K, Y_K, Z_K respectively, then with assumed accuracy of the dipole
approximation

$$X_K = p_x X_L + q_x Y_L + r_x Z_L$$
$$Y_K = p_y X_L + q_y Y_L + r_y Z_L \qquad (11.2)$$
$$Z_K = p_z X_L + q_z Y_L + r_z Z_L$$

wherein the 9 coefficients $p_x \ldots r_z$ are dimensionless magnitudes, dependent only upon the choice of the coordinate system and system K and L.
In the set of three equations, $X_K \ldots Z_L$ are known while the coefficients
are unknown. If we wish to calculate the latter we must expand the number
of equations to at least nine, i.e., we must establish Eq. (11.2) for at least
three isophasal pairs of points. Instead of three, we can take five points on
the loops and establish equations for each pair. We then have 15 equations
for 9 unknowns. The problem is now overdetermined. In order to solve the
system of equations in such a case we can use the method of least squares.
But we go further and solve not for one loop but collect a series of vectorcardiograms for a great number, e.g., N patients [1]) so that we have $3 \times 5 \times N$
equations for nine unknowns. The method of least squares gives us "average"
values for $p_x \ldots r_z$. (The calculations required can only be done by an
electronic computer.)

---

[1]) Calculations in Utrecht were based on 169 cases, 41 normal individuals and 128
patients with heart defects.

The result, written as:

$$X_{L \to K} = p_{x(L \to K)} X_L + q_{x(L \to K)} Y_L + r_{x(L \to K)} Z_L$$
$$Y_{L \to K} = p_{y(L \to K)} X_L + q_{y(L \to K)} Y_L + r_{y(L \to K)} Z_L \qquad (11.3)$$
$$Z_{L \to K} = p_{z(L \to K)} X_L + q_{z(L \to K)} Y_L + r_{z(L \to K)} Z_L$$

shows with which coefficients we have to multiply the three coefficients of the L system in order, after summing, to obtain average components which we would otherwise be able to obtain "directly" from the K system. In other words, the transformation affords the possibility of simulating on an average the vectorcardiograms of the K system by means of the L system.

Without going into the details of the method, we note here certain results which can be taken as examples: the transformations from the M to the S system and from the B to the M system.

$$X_{M \to S} = +(0.86 \pm 0.010)X_M + (0.01 \pm 0.013)Y_M - (0.09 \pm 0.010)Z_M$$
$$Y_{M \to S} = +(0.01 \pm 0.005)X_M + (0.88 \pm 0.006)Y_M + (0.00 \pm 0.005)Z_M \; (11.4)$$
$$Z_{M \to S} = +(0.21 \pm 0.016)X_M + (0.13 \pm 0.021)Y_M + (1.05 \pm 0.016)Z_M$$

$$X_{B \to M} = +(0.71 \pm 0.013)X_B + (0.22 \pm 0.028)Y_B + (0.24 \pm 0.019)Z_B$$
$$Y_{B \to M} = +(0.05 \pm 0.007)X_B + (0.97 \pm 0.011)Y_B - (0.17 \pm 0.010)Z_B \; (11.5)$$
$$Z_{B \to M} = -(0.39 \pm 0.021)X_B + (0.60 \pm 0.033)Y_B + (0.92 \pm 0.030)Z_B$$

How do we judge such a transformation? Of course we must first ascertain what we expect, or rather what we want to appear. That is, as remarked previously, the identical transformation given by the matrix of coefficients (page 64).

$$\begin{pmatrix} 1 & 0 & 0 \\ 0 & 1 & 0 \\ 0 & 0 & 1 \end{pmatrix} \qquad (11.6)$$

In general the coefficients $p_x \ldots r_z$ do not vary too much from those of the identical transformation (see (11.4) and (11.5)), but for certain individuals the correspondence of (11.4) and (11.5) is poor. Not only can we draw the conclusion from this that the systems are clearly unlike, but it is even possible to obtain an indication wherein the systems differ. So the large coefficient $q_{z(B \to M)}$ in (11.5) indicates that a larger y-component in the B system will correspond to a larger z-component in the M system, or, speaking in geometrical terms, a downward-directed loop in the B system corresponds to a somewhat more backward (or less forward-) directed loop in the M system.

In the calculations that lead to a transformation we have to bear in mind that the "absolute size" of the loop plays a role which becomes evident in the measurement of the coordinates of the points. Just as in electrocardiography, this absolute magnitude is generally unimportant in vectorcardiography. Nevertheless a source of error is concealed here, for the ignoring of differences in magnitude as is the practice in the clinic has no objective analogs. Therefore it is necessary to adapt the scales of the different systems to each other as closely as possible. To that end an average measure of the magnitude of the loop is introduced, characterized by:

$$\bar{H} = \sqrt{\left(\frac{\Sigma X^2}{n} + \frac{\Sigma Y^2}{n} + \frac{\Sigma Z^2}{n}\right)} \tag{11.7}$$

whereby all five points of all N systems are summed ($n = 5N$). For each system we make $\bar{H}$ equal to a previously selected standard (for which the B system is used.) Now we have the possibility of adapting the systems to each other in magnitude by means of a correction factor.

With knowledge of the transformation we have not yet a complete quantitative insight, however, into the measure in which the two systems agree or differ (notwithstanding the fact that such information is implicit in the transformation). For the difference between system L and the system $L \to K$ obtained from L by transformation we therefore define the "distance" which is bridged by the transformation as:

$$(L - L \to K) = \sqrt{\{(X_{L \to K} - X_L)^2 + (Y_{L \to K} - Y_L)^2 + (Z_{L \to K} - Z_L)^2\}} \tag{11.8}$$

wherein

$$
\begin{aligned}
(X_{L \to K} - X_L) &= (p_{x(L \to K)} - 1)X_L + q_{x(L \to K)}Y_L + r_{x(L \to K)}Z_L \\
(Y_{L \to K} - Y_L) &= p_{y(L \to K)}X_L + (q_{y(L \to K)} - 1)Y_L + r_{y(L \to K)}Z_L \\
(Z_{L \to K} - Z_L) &= p_{z(L \to K)}X_L + q_{z(L \to K)}Y_L + (r_{z(L \to K)} - 1)Z_L
\end{aligned} \tag{11.9}
$$

For this distance we obtain an average value by substituting for $X_L{}^2$, $Y_L{}^2$, ... etc. in (11.8), the expressions

$$\frac{\Sigma X_L{}^2}{n}, \quad \frac{\Sigma Y_L{}^2}{n}, \quad \ldots \text{ etc.}$$

which are summed over all $5\ N$ points.

If we then divide by $\bar{H}$, we have the average relative distance δ which makes possible the numerical expression of the difference between two systems:

$$\delta = \frac{(L - L \rightarrow K)}{\sqrt{\left(\dfrac{\Sigma X^2}{n} + \dfrac{\Sigma Y^2}{n} + \dfrac{\Sigma Z^2}{n}\right)}} \qquad (11.10)$$

(no confusion can arise over the denominator which is the same for the two systems).

We can now obtain still antoher expression which states how far the L system transformed to K agrees with the true K system. In other words, how successful we have been in imitating the K system with the L system transformed to K. For this we compare $L \rightarrow K$, with K itself. In a way similar to that above, we determine a relative magnitude for this *deviation* (Δ) of $L \rightarrow K$:

$$\Delta = \frac{\sqrt{\{(X_K - X_{L \rightarrow K})^2 + (Y_K - Y_{L \rightarrow K})^2 + (Z_K - Z_{L \rightarrow K})^2\}}}{\sqrt{\left(\dfrac{\Sigma X^2}{n} + \dfrac{\Sigma Y^2}{n} + \dfrac{\Sigma Z^2}{n}\right)}} \cdot \qquad (11.11)$$

The denominator is equal to $\bar{H}$ as defined in (11.7). In this expression we again substitute for X_K^2 the value $(\Sigma X_K^2)/N$, etc.

We present some numerical examples for values δ and Δ to give an impression of the order of magnitudes.

Transformation	δ	Δ
$B \rightarrow M$	0.35	0.44
$M \rightarrow S$	0.22	0.31

(11.12)

What conclusion can we draw from this concerning the practical value of the transformation? Let us consider what can be learned from δ and Δ in extreme cases.

Ideally $\delta = 0$ and $\Delta = 0$. That is to say, on average there is no difference between systems L and K. The transformation is identical and thus need not be worked out. Furthermore, deviation is zero — an inconceivable situation in practice — that is to say that the results of the L and K system are identical at all times [1]).

---

[1]) The latter does not exist in practice, since no vectorcardiograph is equipped to record two or more systems simultaneously. Since the electric activity of the heart in two successive beats is never entirely the same the deviation introduced by this phenomenon cannot be eliminated.

A small δ with a large Δ must mean that the distance covered by the transformation is small with respect to deviation. It is obvious that then the transformation has no single meaning. This contrasts with the situation in which δ has a specific value and the corresponding Δ is small. The transformation can then be fruitfully applied, to obtain with the electrode placement of one system the results of another system of vectorcardiography.

The table presents values for δ and Δ which do not differ greatly. Being aware of the subjective element concealed in a statement in a case like this with little evidence, we assume here that the transformation is meaningful enough (the reader who is not a physicist be well aware that physics, however exact it may seem as a science, cannot exist without human interpretation. Experimental physics are often only exact between the subjective choice of method and the evaluation of the final result).

This conclusion is supported by what a "subjective comparison" yields. If we compare the transformed system with the system to which it is transformed, then generally the evaluation turns out to be more favorable than when we consider the two original vectorcardiograms. This is demonstrated in (11.13) in which the data with respect to the B and M system are reported.

trans-formation	δ	Δ	comparison	subjective evaluation	
				frontal	horizontal
$B \to M$	0.35	0.44	B with M $B \to M$ with M	6.9 ± 0.1 7.9 ± 0.1	5.8 ± 0.1 6.7 ± 0.1

$$(11.13)$$

Fig. 54 presents several examples taken from actual practice. They are intended to illustrate the above discussion, for which reason satisfactorily tallying cases have been selected.

On page 65 we were concerned with the individual transformation. We calculated coefficients $p_x \ldots r_z$ from five pairs of isophasal points. The deviation in the result (hence the divergence of the transformed system from the system to which it was transformed) appears generally small with respect to distance δ over which the transformation is made, as a result of the fact that the transform matrix is "fitted" to the individual. If we compare δ for a greater number of individual transformations we find — unfortunately — great differences, even to a factor of five between maximum and minimum values. Hence the large Δ in the averaged transformation is not the immediate result of inaccuracy of the dipole approximation (for it is successful for one

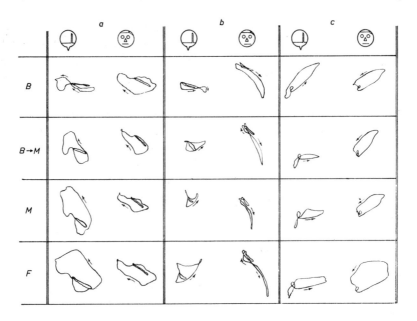

Fig. 54. Three examples of successful transformations from *B* to *M* system

individual) but must stem primarily from the great variations between individuals.

11.3 Conclusions

What can we learn now from all these considerations concerning the comparison of the different systems?

First it has become clear, whatever physical basis has been selected, and whatever hypotheses were developed, there still remains some uncertainty in the final result, because our object is not purely physical in nature but also biological. To conduct electrocardiography by "cook by book recipe" is to blind oneself to the problems involved. Vectorcardiography forces the user to take cognizance of the physical difficulties that are hidden in the method and which only come clearly to light when several systems are used. *Secondly*, each of the four physically based systems which we have considered with few exceptions, leads to the same clinical diagnosis. In this way they can be regarded as clinical equivalents.

The following conclusion is obvious. One system should be selected and applied as the universally accepted one. All the confusion in the field of vectorcardiography would thus be relegated to the past. Comparison of vectorcardiograms made anywhere in the world would be possible.

Unfortunately psychology comes into the discussion when the choice of a system is involved, even to such an extent that what seems to be simple is never brought to fruition.

11.4 Compromise in vectorcardiography

Is physics perhaps in a position to iron out the opposing viewpoints? When differing standpoints must be coordinated, it is usual to hunt for a mutually acceptable compromise. In terms of physics this means that system L ought to be transformed halfway to K, and system K ought to be halfway transformed to L. In practice this can be effected simply by averaging the coefficients. We can average the coefficients of L and those of the transformation of $L \rightarrow K$, in brief notation:

$$L_{LK} = \frac{L + L \rightarrow K}{2} \qquad (11.14)$$

and conversely

$$L_{KL} = \frac{K + K \rightarrow L}{2}. \qquad (11.15)$$

If we compare the two vectorcardiograms which have each undergone a half transformation step according to (11.14) and (11.15), correspondence is certainly better than when a complete transformation is performed. If the users of the two systems L and K would each adjust their respective systems similarly, the results of both operations should be readable without much difficulty although each user is still able to retain his "own" electrode system. To generalize this thought by constructing an "average" system by a transformation of each vectorcardiography system is obvious. If the decision could be made to accept such a proposal, an important step will have been taken in the direction of unified vectorcardiography.

Finally we must address a few comments on the matter of linear transformation. If the average transformation has been calculated to convert system L to system K, the reverse operation from K to L is not yet known.

This can be shown by a one-dimensional case. When a great number of points X_K and X_L is given and an arbitrary point X_L must be transformed to K using $X_{L \to K} = p_{x(L \to K)} X_L$, the method of least squares yields $p_{x(L \to K)}$ through

$$\Sigma X_K X_L = p_{x(L \to K)} \Sigma X_L{}^2. \tag{11.16}$$

For the reverse transformation $X_{K \to L} = p_{x(K \to L)} X_K$ we find $p_{x(K \to L)}$ from

$$\Sigma X_L X_K = p_{x(K \to L)} \Sigma X_K{}^2. \tag{11.17}$$

We see immediately that

$$p_{x(L \to K)} \neq \frac{1}{p_{x(K \to L)}}. \tag{11.18}$$

Unfortunately it is not true that we can deduce the transformation $L_1 \to L_2$ when we know transformations $K \to L_1$ and $K \to L_2$ of three systems, K, L_1 and L_2. This means that we must perform the complete calculation to find the transformation between any pair of systems, and in any direction.

CHAPTER 12

THE POLAR VECTOR (*P*)

Electrocardiography as many other physical techniques, which amass information, provides so much data that one is swanged and unable to see wood for trees. Mathematics long ago divised ways of bringing some comprehensible order into the multiplicity of data by introducing averages, standard deviations, significance tests, etc.

A vectorcardiogram also contains in fact a very great amount of information — no matter how simple the appearance of a loop may be — and we should therefore readily find methods to characterize this information, particularly specific aspects of it, in a simple and visibly striking manner. This wish has led to the introduction of simple magnitudes which are specific for certain properties of the vectorcardiogram. Two of them, *the polar vector* (*P*) and *the ventricular gradient* (*G*) will be discussed in the present and the following chapter respectively.

As we noted previously (page 24) the direction of movement of the dot on the oscilloscope screen at the time of "writing" the vectorcardiogram is an important datum in making a diagnosis. This is especially true of the frontal projection. By using periodic beam interruption it is possible to determine this direction on the record (see Fig. 55): by depression of the electron beam the intensity is diminished little by little so that the "point" of the dot indicates the direction of travel (see footnote page 24). Difficulties arise, however, in that in the frontal projection the loop is seen "on edge". A very flat loop is then developed, rather than an open one, or a figure eight in which one part moves clockwise and the other counterclockwise. The desire to have a clear criterion in such cases also, wherein direction of movement of the vector or, more generally, the spatial orientation of the

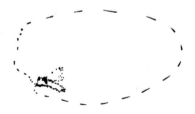

Fig. 55. A vectorcardiogram with time marking. The direction of travel follows from the form of the dots.

plane of the loop is discounted, has been the occasion for the introduction of the "polar vector" concept.

Let us start with the assumption that the loop (we always mean that of the QRS complex) lies entirely in a flat plane. We indicate the orientation of this plane by the normal vector thereon. The direction of this normal vector is the same as that in which a right-handed screw would advance when turned in the sense in which the VCG is written. The particular feature that we want to characterize can thus easily be expressed by the position of this "*polar vector*" (= normal vector).

It seems less simple to find a similar criterion for the case in which the loop is not in a flat plane but twists arbitrarily through space. As we shall prove, it is still possible in that case to define a polar vector.

Through the closed curve — as the QRS loop of a vectorcardiogram usually is — we provide an arbitrarily curved surface (S). By means of it we are able to determine a definition of the normal vector of the "surface of the loop". We divide S into surface elements dS which are so small that we may consider each individually as a plane. Each of these elements can be represented by a vector, perpendicular on and with a length proportional to its area and pointing in a direction which, as we indicated above, follows from the law of the right-hand screw applied to the vectorcardiogram. All vectors that we can construct in this way are added. This vector sum is then P. Within the limit this becomes an integral:

$$\int dS = P. \tag{12.1}$$

We shall show that this expression is not dependent upon the choice of the supplied surface, but is exclusively determined by the contour thereof, hence by the vectorcardiogram. We supply a second surface S' through the curve, so that a sort of lenticular enclosure is developed. We also divide S' into elements to develop $\int dS'$ in analogy to (12.1) on the understanding that we oppose the direction of dS' on S' to the direction of dS on S.

If we inquire about the sum of the two integrals, we encounter a known fact: the vector integral of the superficial elements of a closed surface is zero (see note on page 71). Thus for *unidirectional* dS and dS':

$$\int dS = \int dS' = P. \tag{12.2}$$

P is thus exclusively dependent upon the contour of the surface, hence upon the vectorcardiogram.

How do we determine P in practice? It can be done very simply, because the three components of P are exactly equal to the area of the corresponding projection of the vectorcardiogram. It can be readily seen that this is true for a flat surface because the area of the projection on the y,z-plane and P_x are both determined by multiplying the surface and P respectively by $cos\ \alpha$, whereby α is the same in both cases. That the statement is also valid for a curved surface is a consequence of the fact that we can think of it as composed of small flat surfaces.

The areas of the three projections are determined by means of a planimeter. With this in view, it is important that the vectorcardiograph should have three oscilloscope screens.

As already mentioned experience has shown that diagnostically the magnitude of the loop has less significance than *the orientation of the loop in space* and the direction in which it moves. This has led to the following geometric representation and clinical technique. We cause the pole vector to originate in the center of a sphere (of any radius). The point where this sphere is intersected by P precisely characterizes the information wherewith clinical practice deals. For practical execution the cartesian coordinates x, y and z must of course be transformed to polar coordinates r, φ and ϑ of which only the latter two are used to determine azimuth and elevation on the sphere.

So we can determine the orientation of the QRS-complex plane of the vectorcardiogram for a great number of patients and join the diagnosis to the point of intersection of P with the sphere (the diagnosis being obtained of course *without* this datum). It then appears that for specific pathological cases these points of intersection are found in a more or less demarcated part of the sphere surface which is characteristic for the specific disease while other diseases in this respect show no preference. Up to this point the atrial septal defect is a very characteristic example: the two types are distinguished by diametral polar vector positions (see page 132).

CHAPTER 13

THE VENTRICULAR GRADIENT (*G*)

In the previous chapter we showed how the polar vector *P* was introduced to determine *the orientation of the surface of the vectorcardiogram in space.*

Another similar magnitude which also reveals a property of the loop in its entirety can be found in *the averaged direction of the heart vector H(t).* This magnitude is designated *the ventricular gradient (G).* That *G* is essentially something other than *P* can be seen from Fig. 56, wherein the schematically drawn curves can be thought to be in a plane and therefore all have the same *P* direction but different *G* (it is also possible to alter the position (hence *P*) of for example, loop 1 by rotation about *G₁* as axis, without changing the ventricular gradient in any way).

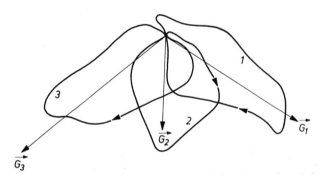

Fig. 56. Three vectorcardiograms on one single plane, being characterised by one and the same **P**, but with different **G**

We can furnish an unequivocal formula for *G*:

$$G = \int H(t)\,dt. \tag{13.1}$$

Here we can perceive an expansion of the time integral which was developed in electrocardiography of $V(t)$ (the electrocardiogram).

Formula (13.1) can be applied during the depolarization period (the *QRS* complex), the repolarization period (*T*) or both in combination. In the latter case:

$$G_{QRS,T} = G_{QRS} + G_T. \tag{13.2}$$

The action of the atria (P wave of the electrocardiogram) is not included because the integral of depolarization and repolarization yields a value for it which can be neglected.

No agreement has been reached concerning the diagnostic significance of G. Insofar as it is of clinical value, this value derives from the fact that G is regarded as being independent of the origin of excitation in the heart. As such it could be an indication of the state of the myocardium.

G's independence of the location of excitation, postulated in the past, can be made plausible by a simple general hypothesis.

We assume the myocardium to be a volume of any conformation (Fig. 57). At a given instant, we assume, a part of the muscle will be excited (the hatched portion in Fig. 57), while the rest is still in polarised state (see page 16). The boundary surface between the two areas is a thin layer that runs through the heart as an (excitation) front (we will return to a discussion of this excitation front in Chapter 15).

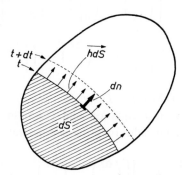

Fig. 57. The excitation front of the heart at time t and $t + dt$. The part excited at t is hatched

A general description of the excitation front may be given by the equation of a plane moving in time:

$$F(x,y,z,t) = 0 \qquad (13.3)$$

in which x, y and z are orthogonal coordinates and t is the time. We can assume a solution for t from this expression. How this is to be done is not important for the rest of the calculation. We here only give t generally as a function of x, y and z

$$t = f(x,y,z). \qquad (13.4)$$

Because it will be assumed that the boundary surface F is the place where the source of electric heart action is seated, the "origin" therefore of the local heart vector (see Chapter 15), we see F as a dipole layer. In Fig. 57 this is indicated by arrows standing perpendicular to the layer. Each arrow represents the contribution $h\mathrm{d}S$ of the dipole effect of a surface element $\mathrm{d}S$. All arrows together constitute the heart vector. If we assume that the dipole contribution to H of each surface element $\mathrm{d}S$ is proportional to the area of that element, H can be found by the surface integral

$$H = \int_S h\mathrm{d}S \tag{13.5}$$

wherein $|h|$ for the entire myocardium is assumed to be constant. In time interval $\mathrm{d}t$ the front will have moved over distance $\mathrm{d}n$ (which does not need to be uniform everywhere) (Fig. 57). By means of elementary analysis we can state that

$$\mathrm{d}n = \frac{\mathrm{d}t}{\left[\left(\frac{\partial t}{\partial x}\right)^2 + \left(\frac{\partial t}{\partial y}\right)^2 + \left(\frac{\partial t}{\partial z}\right)^2\right]^{1/2}} \tag{13.6}$$

or

$$\mathrm{d}t = \mathrm{d}n \left[\left(\frac{\partial t}{\partial x}\right)^2 + \left(\frac{\partial t}{\partial y}\right)^2 + \left(\frac{\partial t}{\partial z}\right)^2\right]^{1/2} \tag{13.7}$$

wherein according to (13.4), $t = f(x,y,z)$.

If we substitute this last equation and (13.5) in (13.1), we obtain (if for the time being we consider only the depolarization)

$$G_{QRS} = \int_n \left[\int_S h\mathrm{d}S\right]\left[\left(\frac{\partial t}{\partial x}\right)^2 + \left(\frac{\partial t}{\partial y}\right)^2 + \left(\frac{\partial t}{\partial z}\right)^2\right]^{1/2} \mathrm{d}n. \tag{13.8}$$

Because $\mathrm{d}S\mathrm{d}n = \mathrm{d}v$, a volume element of the myocardium, (13.8) goes over into

$$G_{QRS} = \int_{vol} h\left[\left(\frac{\partial t}{\partial x}\right)^2 + \left(\frac{\partial t}{\partial y}\right)^2 + \left(\frac{\partial t}{\partial z}\right)^2\right]^{1/2} \mathrm{d}v. \tag{13.9}$$

The expression between square brackets can be rewritten. It is a well known fact, that (see Eq. (13.4))

$$\left(\frac{\partial t}{\partial x}, \frac{\partial t}{\partial y}, \frac{\partial t}{\partial z}\right) = \mathbf{grad}\, f = \nabla f. \tag{13.10}$$

The absolute value of this vector is given by

$$\left[\left(\frac{\partial t}{\partial x}\right)^2 + \left(\frac{\partial t}{\partial y}\right)^2 + \left(\frac{\partial t}{\partial z}\right)^2\right]^{1/2} = |\nabla f|. \tag{13.11}$$

If we recall that ∇f has the direction of dn, the normal vector of the surface of excitation, and that moreover h is directed along this normal, then using $h = |h|$ we can write for (13.9)

$$G_{QRS} = \int_{\text{vol}} h \, |\nabla f| \, dv = h \int_{\text{vol}} \nabla f \, dv. \tag{13.12}$$

Some time after the excitation a recovery process (repolarization) will extend over the heart. We assume that this repolarization occurs at time τ after depolarization. Because this time interval is not the same for all parts of the myocardium, τ shall be a function of the coordinates: $\tau = \tau(x,y,z)$.

If we now wish to solve (13.1) for repolarization we must fill in for the time

$$t + \tau = f(x,y,z) + \tau(x,y,z). \tag{13.13}$$

Since the rest of the calculation proceeds similarly we mention only the result

$$G_T = \int_T H(t) dt = -h \int_{\text{vol}} (\nabla f + \nabla \tau) \, dv \tag{13.14}$$

in which the minus sign appears because in repolarization h has the opposite direction with respect to the area over which we now integrate.

According to (13.2) we have to add (13.12) and (13.14) to determine the total $G_{QRS,T}$:

$$G_{QRS,T} = G_{QRS} + G_T = \int H(t) \, dt = -h \int_{\text{vol}} \nabla \tau \, dv. \tag{13.15}$$

It is shown hereby, with the acceptance of simple general hypothesis, that the ventricular gradient is independent of the way in which excitation passes through the heart. At the same time (13.15) gives meaning to the word *"gradient"* which previously was selected without this background. This $\nabla \tau$ results, as already noted, from the fact that the time interval between de-polarization and repolarization differs from one location to another.

It is not precisely understood how this $\nabla \tau$ occurs. It has been suggested that it relates to a temperature gradient but there is no certainty about this.

If we compare the polar vector (*P*) and ventricular gradient (*G*), obviously *G* may be represented geometrically in the same way as *P*, i.e., we take the center of a sphere as the origin of *G* and find the place where the vector intersects the sphere (thereby again shifting the data concerning the length of *G*). We can, with the aid of *P* and *G* determine two points on the sphere surface for each loop and with this pair of points the *QRS* loop of the vectorcardiogram is acceptably characterized.

We can now apply statistics on the point distribution on the sphere, in order to obtain data concerning specific pathological conditions.

Rather than go into details we indicate the following: it will be clear that the ventricular gradient implicitly includes time, in contrast to vector *P* which depends only on the spatial orientation of the surface and not upon the way in which — in time — the loop is traced. The table below shows the situation clearly:

	with *t*	without *t*
P		+
G	+	

We may ask about the possibility of determining more general expressions for the two magnitudes, thus filling in the blanks in the diagram. It appears to be possible indeed.

We will not go further into the solution of this problem. Suffice it to say that probably with computers it may be possible to obtain valuable diagnostic data from the results.

In this connection it should be possible to find still one more datum in determining the direction (and possibly the magnitude) of the heart vector after a specific time interval of *t* milliseconds after its "start" (for the total time scale this comes near to the explicit determination of the way in which the loop is traced in time). This "*t*-millisecond vector" can again be characterized by the point of intersection with a sphere. Without doubt, provided the value of *t* is suitably selected, the distribution of the points on the sphere would yield valuable information in distinguishing specific types of heart diseases. Experiments, for the frontal projection only, have already been performed (a circle then replaces the sphere) and not without success. Attacking the problem of the 3-dimensional case is decidedly worthwhile.

CHAPTER 14

THE MULTIPOLE EFFECT

14.1 General theory

In our consideration of the heart vector we have so far dealt exclusively with the dipole effect, ignoring the contribution of higher poles. Only in passing (page 29) did we indicate that the potential at a point P caused by a cluster of single poles, positive as well as negative, in a homogeneous medium can be described as the sum of the monopole, dipole, quadrupole, ... effect:

$$V_P = \frac{\Phi_1}{r} + \frac{\Phi_2}{r^2} + \frac{\Phi_3}{r^3} + \ldots . \tag{5.18}$$

The requirement for rapid convergence of the series and the fact that the first term was assumed to be zero, made us set the potential as equal to the second term. In this chapter however we shall go somewhat more deeply into the general theory of potentials, in connection with Chapter 5 in order to examine to what extend higher poles contribute to the expression for the potential. We shall pay special attention to the quadrupole.

We first consider the series (5.18) in more detail. We consider a cluster of point sources I_i within a small region of a homogeneous infinitely extended medium. The distance of each source from the origin O of a system of coordinates, provisionally random among the point sources, we designate r_i (Fig. 58). The potential V_P at a point P, distance r from O, and distance R_i from I_i can be expressed, if we also assume

$$\frac{I_i}{4\pi\sigma} \equiv q_i,$$

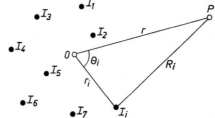

Fig. 58. In the calculation of the potential at a point P, outside a cluster of point sources

by the equation:

$$V_P = \sum_i \frac{q_i}{R_i}.$$ (14.1)

We shall convert this expression. Substituting the cosine rule:

$$R_i^2 = r^2 + r_i^2 - 2rr_i \cos \theta_i$$ (14.2)

in (14.1) we have for V_P:

$$V_P = \sum_i \frac{q_i}{(r^2 + r_i^2 - 2rr_i \cos \theta_i)^{1/2}}$$

or

$$V_P = \sum_i \frac{q_i}{r} \left[1 + \left(\frac{r_i}{r} \right)^2 - 2 \frac{r_i}{r} \cos \theta_i \right]^{-1/2},$$ (14.3)

Although it may be assumed to be generally known that an expression in Legendre polynomials can be used for (14.3) we will go into the matter briefly. Formula (14.3) has the form

$$F(x,y) = (1 + y^2 - 2xy)^{-1/2}$$ (14.4)

This function can be developed in a series, as we shall show briefly. If $F(x,y)$ is differentiated n times according to y at point $y = 0$, the result is:

$$\left(\frac{d^n F(x,y)}{dy^n} \right)_{y=0} = l! \, P_l(x)$$ (14.5)

where $P_l(x)$ are Legendre polynomials:

$$P_0 = 1, \quad P_1 = x, \quad P_2 = \tfrac{1}{2}(3x^2 - 1), \quad P_3 = \tfrac{1}{2}(5x^3 - 3x), \ldots.$$

If we develop $F(x,y)$ at $y = 0$, we get

$$F(x,y) = F(x,0) + y \left(\frac{\partial F}{\partial y} \right)_{y=0} + \frac{y^2}{2!} \left(\frac{\partial^2 F}{\partial y^2} \right)_{y=0} + \ldots + \frac{y^l}{l!} \left(\frac{\partial^l F}{\partial y^l} \right)_{y=0}$$ (14.6)

Applying (14.5), this becomes:

$$F(x,y) = (1 + y^2 - 2xy)^{-1/2} = \sum_l y^l P_l(x)$$ (14.7)

We can only apply this expression as the right hand member converges, which will be the case when $y < 1$ and $P_l(x) \leqslant 1$. It is possible to show that the latter is true when $|x| \leqslant 1$.

The general expression (14.7) is applied to the potential equation (14.3). This equation then becomes:

$$V_P = \sum_i \frac{q_i}{r} \sum_l \left(\frac{r_i}{r}\right)^l P_l (\cos \theta_i) \qquad (14.8)$$

or

$$V_P = \sum_l \frac{\sum_i q_i r_i{}^l P_l(\cos \theta_i)}{r^{l+1}}. \qquad (14.9)$$

When point P is far enough outside the clustered sources, then $r_i/r < 1$ so that conditions for convergence of the series are fulfilled. If we now designate:

$$\sum_i q_i r_i{}^l P_l (\cos \theta_i) \equiv Q_l \qquad (14.10)$$

we have a simple expression for the multipole development:

$$V_P = \sum_l \frac{Q_l}{r^{l+1}} \qquad (14.11)$$

wherein Q_l is independent of r. In our case, since as much electricity flows out from every volume element of the heart as comes in, the term for the single pole is discarded, so that:

$$Q_0 = \sum_i q_i = \frac{1}{4\pi\sigma} \sum_i I_i = 0.$$

We shall now clarify this theory by some examples.

14.2 Examples

14.2.1. We consider a current doublet. The origin of the system of coordinates is chosen in the middle, between the $+$ and $-$ poles. We calculate the potential at a point P and distance r from 0 (Fig. 59) by means of (14.11) and (14.10). If the data of Fig. 59 are substituted in these formulae, taking into account of the current by sign, and recalling that the angle between r and $r-$ is equal to $\theta + \pi$, and with consideration that $|r_+| = |r_-| = U$, it

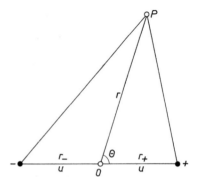

Fig. 59. A current doublet with origin of the system of coordinates halfway between the poles

is easy to understand that

$$V_P = \frac{2I}{4\pi\sigma}\left(\frac{UP_1\,(\cos\theta)}{r^2} + \frac{U^3P_3\,(\cos\theta)}{r^4} + \ldots\right). \qquad (14.12)$$

The first term is the — anticipated — dipole component, and the second term represents the octapole effect. *We see that the quadrupole term is absent.* As will be seen later, this is due to the choice of position of the origin.

14.2.2. As second example, we choose a so-called dipole shell. This is a circular disc (radius a) whose midpoint coincides with the origin of our system of coordinates and which has a balanced dipole distribution so that the right side of the disc contains the positive pole and the left side of it the negative (Fig. 60) (in fact we meet here a special case of a dipole shell) (see also Chapter 15). We again calculate the potential at point P, distance r from O. We take into consideration only the case $r > a$. For reasons of symmetry V_P must be a function of r and θ. Since this function — which we again write as a series — must be finite for $r \to \infty$, the series will contain only negative powers of r. Since $P_l \cos\theta \,/\, r^{l+1}$ satisfies the Laplace

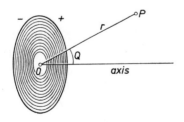

Fig. 60. A homogeneous dipole shell

equation ($\nabla^2 V = 0$), we may write for V_P in analogy to (14.11)

$$V_P = b_1 \frac{P_1 \cos \theta}{r^2} + b_2 \frac{P_2 \cos \theta}{r^3} + b_3 \frac{P_3 \cos \theta}{r^4} + \ldots \quad (14.13)$$

It is possible to determine the constant factors b_i by calculating the potential for the special case of a point on the axis. We shall perform this calculation. Because for any point on the axis, $\theta = 0$ and therefore $P_i \cos \theta = P_i \cos 0 = P_i(1) = 1$, the potential in a point on the axis at distance r from the origin must satisfy

$$V_{\text{axis}} = \frac{b_1}{r^2} + \frac{b_2}{r^3} + \frac{b_3}{r^4} + \ldots \quad (14.14)$$

V_{axis} can also be calculated by solving the integral $\int_\Omega V \, dS$, in which

$$V \, dS = \frac{dD \cos \varphi}{4\pi s^2} \, dS. \quad (14.15)$$

Ω is the area of the circular dipole shell, and dS is a surface element of it.

In Eq. (14.15) D is the total dipole moment of the disk, dD thus is the dipole strength per area thereof, s is the distance of the surface element dS to point Q on the axis, distance r from O and φ the angle as defined earlier (see Fig. 61, compare Fig. 18 and Eq. (5.17) page 29) (Note that φ in Eq. (14.15) has the same meaning as had θ in (5.17)).

When we take the surface element dS annular, then (see Fig. 61)

$$dD \, dS = \frac{D}{\pi a^2} 2\pi \varrho \, d\varrho$$

whereas

$$s = (\varrho^2 + r^2)^{1/2}.$$

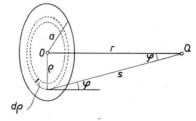

Fig. 61. In the calculation of the potential at a point Q at distance r from a homogeneous dipole shell

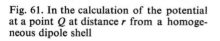

Now V_{axis} becomes:

$$V_{\text{axis}} = \int_{\varrho=0}^{a} \frac{D}{\pi a^2} \, 2\pi\varrho \, d\varrho \, \frac{1}{4\pi(r^2 + \varrho^2)} \frac{r}{(r^2 + \varrho^2)^{1/2}}. \qquad (14.16)$$

Calculation of the integral yields

$$V_{\text{axis}} = \frac{Dr}{4\pi a^2} \, 2 \left[r^{-1} - (a^2 + r^2)^{-1/2} \right]. \qquad (14.17)$$

To compare this expression with (14.14) we write it as a series

$$V_{\text{axis}} = \frac{D}{4\pi a^2} \left(\frac{a^2}{r^2} - \frac{3}{2 \cdot 2!} \frac{a^4}{r^4} + \frac{3 \cdot 5}{2^2 \cdot 3!} \frac{a^6}{r^6} - \cdots \right). \qquad (14.18)$$

Comparison of Eq. (14.18) with Eq. (14.14) yields for the constant coefficients b_i:

$$b_1 = \frac{D}{4\pi}, \quad b_2 = 0, \quad b_3 = \frac{D}{4\pi} \frac{3}{4} a^2, \quad b_4 = 0, \quad b_5 = \frac{D}{4\pi} \frac{15}{24} a^3, \quad \text{etc.}$$

Substituting these values in (14.13) yields:

$$V_P = \frac{D}{4\pi r^2} \left[P_1 \cos\theta - \frac{3}{4} \frac{a^2}{r^2} P_3 \cos\theta + \frac{5}{8} \frac{a^4}{r^4} P_5 \cos\theta - \cdots \right]. \qquad (14.19)$$

The first term is again the dipole effect, the second the octapole component etc. *It is striking that the quadrupole, like all other terms with odd powers of r, is again missing.*

14.2.3. In the following example the origin of the system of coordinates is placed at an arbitrary point on the connecting line between two current poles I and $-I$, combined to form a current doublet (Fig. 62) (in the limit $(r_1 - r_2) \to 0$ the doublet again goes over into a dipole.) It is again readily seen (see example 14.2.1) that the potential at a point P at distance r from O must satisfy (for the meaning of r_1 and r_2, see Fig. 62)

$$V_P = \frac{I}{4\pi\sigma} \left[\frac{r_1 - r_2}{r^2} P_1 \cos\theta + \frac{r_1{}^2 - r_2{}^2}{r^3} P_2 \cos\theta + \frac{r_1{}^3 - r_2{}^3}{r^4} P_3 \cos\theta + \cdots \right]$$

$$(14.20)$$

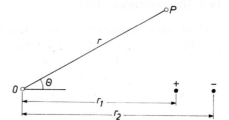

Fig. 62. The origin at an arbitrary point
on the axis of a current doublet

In this case the quadrupole term appears to be present. In view of the fact
that this was not the case in the first example, *the presence of the quadrupole
term must be explained by the choice of the origin of the system of coordinates*,
since we did not use a possible different position of P with reference to the
doublet. In general we may say that the shift in position of the origin has
no effect on the dipole, but it does have it on higher poles.

14.2.4. Finally we take not one but rather two different current doublets.
For the sake of simplicity we assume that at all poles the same current I is
introduced or conducted away and that the difference in the doublet strength
will be determined by the mutual distance of the poles. Somewhere on the
line on which the poles are assumed to lie (Fig. 63) we select the origin.
The potential at P is again calculated by application of (14.10) and (14.11)

$$V_P = \frac{I}{4\pi\sigma}\left[\frac{P_1\cos\theta}{r^2}(r_1-r_2-r_3+r_4) + \frac{P_2\cos\theta}{r^3}(r_1{}^2-r_2{}^2+r_3{}^2-r_4{}^2) + ..\right].$$

(14.21)

The presence of the quadrupole term is now not only a consequence of the
choice of the origin but also of the fact that here we have an intrinsic quadrupole.

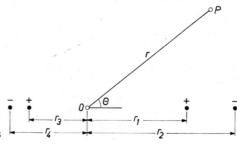

Fig. 63. Two different current doublets

14.3 The quadrupole effect

From these examples we have learned that in the expression for the potential in any point at a certain distance from a cluster of poles, the quadrupole component is dependent upon the position of the origin of our coordinate system. Therefore we can now ask ourselves how far it is possible to make the quadrupole component minimal by an appropriate choice of this origin. Then, perhaps it would be possible in vectorcardiography to get around the difficulties that result from the fact that the dipole approximation is not exactly correct, as we indicated in earlier chapters. It will be immediately understood that it is possible to effect this. If we shift the origin by a distance δ we can write for $r_1{}^2 - r_2{}^2$ in the quadrupole term in (14.20): $(r_1 + \delta)^2 - (r_2 + \delta)^2$. If the quadrupole is to disappear, then:

$$(r_1 + \delta)^2 - (r_2 + \delta)^2 = 0 \quad . \tag{14.22}$$

From this condition it follows for δ that

$$\delta = -\tfrac{1}{2}(r_1 + r_2). \tag{14.23}$$

In reality, however, the origin can become so far removed from the heart, even from the human body, that it becomes a physical impossibility *while the intrinsic quadrupole can never be eliminated*. Although in medical circles suggestions can be heard for the setting up of investigations into these problems, we believe that no meaningful practical progress can be anticipated from them.

It would be better to assign the coordinates system its origin in the "midpoint" of the heart, in order experimentally to determine the magnitudes that characterize the quadrupole effect.

Before we go into this more deeply, we return to theory. We saw in (14.11) how the potential at a point P, caused by a cluster of sources, could be expressed by a series in negative powers of r. We shall write this series in a somewhat different form by using spherical polar rather than cartesian coordinates for the description of point P (Fig. 58). Consequently the formalism of Q_l must be adopted: Now Q_l becomes a function of azimuth and elevation of the radius vector at P.

Instead of Q_l we now write Φ_n and take $n = i + l$, to make the index of Φ agree with the power of r. (We are not going into the explicit form of Φ_n, because it is of no interest in the following consideration.) Thus

$$V_P = \sum_{n=1} \frac{\Phi_n}{r^n} = \frac{\Phi_1}{r} + \frac{\Phi_2}{r^2} + \frac{\Phi_3}{r^3} + \dots \; . \tag{5.18}$$

We have thus recovered the first statement of the series (see (5.18) page 103 and page 30).

There appears to be a practical advantage when we introduce still another formalism, that is a combination of cartesian and spherical polar coordinates. This can be done by means of (5.18). We return to the single dipole (page 29). We saw there that for the potential at a point P at distance r from the dipole

$$V_P (:) \frac{\cos \theta}{r^2} . \tag{14.24}$$

If we multiply numerator and denominator by r, so

$$V_P (:) \frac{r \cos \theta}{r^3} \tag{14.25}$$

then $r \cos \theta$ can be conceived to be the carthesian x-coordinate. Since Φ_n as we observed, is a function of the direction cosine at P, we can attempt to generalize it by writing the term for the dipole of (5.18):

$$\frac{\Phi_2}{r^2} = \frac{r\Phi_2}{r^3} \tag{14.26}$$

and considering whether it is generally possible to substitute

$$V_{P(\text{dipole})} = \frac{r\Phi_2}{r^3} = \frac{ax + by + cz}{r^3} \tag{14.27}$$

wherein x, y and z are the customary cartesian coordinates and a, b and c are determined by the dipole strength. It is easily proved that (14.27) indeed satisfies the Laplace equation $\nabla^2 V = 0$.

A similar operation applied to the *quadrupole* term entails investigation of the permissibility of writing

$$V_{P(\text{quadrupole})} = \frac{r^2 \Phi_3}{r^5} = \frac{kx^2 + ly^2 + mz^2 + syz + txz + uxy}{r^5} . \tag{14.28}$$

It appears that this expression satisfies Laplace, though upon condition that

$$k + l + m = 0. \tag{14.29}$$

Similar expressions can also be found for higher poles which, again under certain conditions, satisfy $\nabla^2 V = 0$. We shall not go any farther into this.

We see by these simple ways of formulating (14.26) and (14.27) — simple because complex generalized Legendre functions are disposed with — that the dipole, as we anticipated, is given by three magnitudes which correspond to the three vector components of the dipole moment. The quadrupole term consists of six magnitudes, k, l, m, s, t and u. However, the extra relation between the first three makes it so that the quadrupole field is characterized not by six magnitudes but rather by $6 - 1 = 5$.

We speak here of a tensor (here a tensor of the second order, because we designate a tensor of the first order as a vector. A vector and a tensor are distinguished by the way in which they are transformed by rotation of the coordinate system. The components of a vector transformed by rotation are linear functions of the direction cosines which determine the rotation, while in the same case a tensor of the second order is quadratically transformed).

From the above we see that if we are not satisfied in "vector"-cardiography with the vectorial dipole effect but also take the quadrupole components into account, we must solve for five extra unknowns simultaneously! But then the previous minimum of four electrodes is no longer sufficient. The $3 + 5 = 8$ independent data which we now have to determine require 8 independent leads, hence at least 9 electrodes (by which we do not mean to say that any number of electrodes greater than four would not be meaningful in "classic" vectorcardiography. The contrary is true, as appears from Chapter 10).

We shall briefly mention how technique can be adapted to this. We again follow the procedure that we applied earlier (page 35). We write the difference of potential between a certain electrode somewhere on the body surface and a reference electrode (which of course may also be located on the body surface) as a linear combination of the 3 dipole and 5 quadrupole components

$$V_{P_1} - V_{P_0} = V_1 = a_1 X + b_1 Y + c_1 Z + d_1 Q_1 +$$
$$+ e_1 Q_2 + f_1 Q_3 + g_1 Q_4 + h_1 Q_5 \quad (14.30)$$

The 8 coefficients $a_1 \ldots h_1$ can be found by model experiments, analogous to those described earlier (Chapter 8) with respect to the "lead vectors". We now find not only a lead vector ($\mathbf{abc}$) but at the same time a lead tensor ($\mathfrak{defgh}$).

If we do this for 8 different pairs of electrodes

$$V_{P_1} - V_{P_0} = V_1 = a_1 X + b_1 Y + c_1 Z + d_1 Q_1 + e_1 Q_2 + f_1 Q_3 + g_1 Q_4 + h_1 Q_5$$

$$V_{P_2} - V_{P_0} = V_2 =$$

$$V_{P_8} - V_{P_0} = V_8 = a_8 X + b_8 Y + c_8 z + d_8 Q_1 + e_8 Q_2 + f_8 Q_3 + g_8 Q_4 + h_8 Q_5$$

$$(14.31)$$

and determine 64 constants $a_1 \ldots h_8$ on the model, then conversely we can find the 8 components which describe the electric activity of the heart (see page 35), using differences of potential measured on the human body.

$$
\begin{aligned}
X &= \alpha_1 V_1 + \alpha_2 V_2 + \alpha_3 V_3 + \alpha_4 V_4 + \alpha_5 V_5 + \alpha_6 V_6 + \alpha_7 V_7 + \alpha_8 V_8 \\
Y &= \beta_1 V_1 + \\
Z &= \gamma_1 V_1 + \\
Q_1 &= \delta_1 V_1 + \\
Q_2 &= \varepsilon_1 V_1 + \\
Q_3 &= \zeta_1 V_1 + \\
Q_4 &= \eta_1 V_1 + \\
Q_5 &= \vartheta_1 V_1 + \vartheta_2 V_2 + \vartheta_3 V_3 + \vartheta_4 V_4 + \vartheta_5 V_5 + \vartheta_6 V_6 + \vartheta_7 V_7 + \vartheta_8 V_8
\end{aligned}
$$

$$(14.32)$$

Instead of 8 voltages, we can select 9, 10, ... The problem which is now overdetermined, can be solved by application of the method of least squares (and an electronic computer) (octapoles and higher poles are neglected).

Of course it is not possible to join the five quadrupole components in one single figure, as the vectorcardiogram brings into the picture the behaviour of the dipole vector during the heart cycle. We can do no more than record the Q's as five separate time functions and take into account these curves in the consideration that lead to the diagnosis of the heart being examined.

With this technique we revert to a certain extent to electrocardiography. However, the method here expounded, although it may seem simple is so complex and hence so uncertain in experimental results that clinical applications are rare.

CHAPTER 15

THE ORIGIN OF THE ELECTRICAL ACTIVITY
OF THE HEART

15.1 General

In all that we have said so far concerning the electrical activity of the heart we have avoided discussing the phenomena that may be considered responsible for this activity. It is the purpose of this chapter to deal with this subject. It should be emphasized that no exhaustive treatment is contemplated. We will content ourselves with a broad outline appropriate to this essay and adequate to provide a foundation for the main object of our study.

We have seen that the representation of the electrical activity of the heart using a single dipole, stationary with respect to place, yields no truly satisfactory result. In Chapters 13 and 14 we used another approach which will prove to be more realistic, by introducing the concept of the excitation front (dipole front or dipole shell). This approach is arisen from measurements of potential at the surface of the heart. Fig. 64 shows how the excitation front may be conceived. This shows a section of the heart, one portion of which is excited (the hatched portion) while the rest is conversely at rest. The electrical dipole effect is directed from the excited part to the non-excited part.

More refined measurement techniques in later years, whereby measurements can be made in the myocardium, have confirmed and extended hypo-

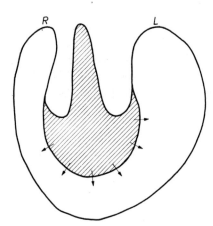

Fig. 64. Diagrammatic section of the heart with excitation front

theses concerning the excitation front. As a preface to the results of these experiments we will describe certain details of the techniques employed.

To penetrate the heart a probe is required equipped with electrodes. A fine hollow needle has been used which has small apertures (0.1 mm in diameter) over part of its length. These openings, which are spaced at distances of the order of 1 millimeter apart, contain the outer ends of wires that are bundled into the needle: thus comprising a system of microelectrodes between each pair of which the voltage can be measured. If one or more of these needles is thrust into the heart (systems with up to 21 needles have been used) it is possible by measuring the voltages between the electrodes as a function of time to get an impression of the properties of the excitation front.

Use may be made of the bipolar or of the unipolar methods. In the latter the voltage is measured between the needle electrodes and a fixed electrode placed, for example, somewhere on the body while in the former case voltages between adjacent pairs of electrodes in the needle are measured. The course of the potential as it appears in the two systems when the excitation front passes an electrode is schematically shown in Fig. 65.

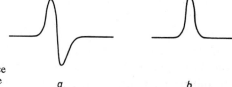

Fig. 65. *a*) Characteristic unipolar trace
         b) Characteristic bipolar trace   *a*   *b*

From the distance separating the electrodes in the needle, the difference in time between the same phenomena in the successive electrodes and the form of the curves, the speed of propagation of the front and the thickness of the excited layer can be measured. The thickness of the excitation front is found to be no more than 1 mm. In relation to the thickness of the myocardium this is so thin that we can speak of a true dipole shell.

Different values have been obtained for the speed of propagation in different tissues, thus:

        Myocardium (heart muscle)   30 to   50 cm/s
        Purkinje (stimulus conducting) tissue   100 to 170 cm/s
        Atrioventricular node   5 to   12 cm/s

The first two values relate to the QRS complex, hence to the contraction phase of the ventricles (the electrical phenomena occurring in the recovery process appear to be less readily measurable). The results agree with what we might expect from the electrocardiogram, where the *QRS* complex is accomplished in about 100 ms. (If the relevant heart dimension is about 10 cm and the propagation speed is 140 cm/s, then the duration of travel of the stimulus through the conducting system is derived as 10/140 s $\approx$ 70 ms. To this the time has to be added required for the impulse to traverse the thickness of the muscle: 1/30 s $\approx$ 30 ms.)

We would draw special attention to the low speed at which the excitation is conducted in the tissue comprising the atrioventricular node. It is here that the delay occurs between the stimulation of the atria and the ventricles which causes the latter to contract *after* the former have completed their contraction, thus producing an efficient ejection.

15.2 Histology of the heart

How can we derive the dipole front from the microstructure of the myo-cardium? Like other muscles, the myocardium consists of fibres which vary in thickness from 30 to 100 μm. The fibres are the living cells themselves [1]).

The muscular tissue of the myocardium is striated, as is that of the skeletal muscles; it differs from the skeletal musculature, however, in that the fibres are ramified and interconnected. Cutting across the three-dimensional net-work thus formed divisions are seen that can be considered to be the cell boundaries (intercalated discs). Per cell one to a few nuclei occur (Fig. 66).

Capillaries supplied by the coronary arteries run in the interstices. In skeletal muscle the fibres do not branch and each fibre contains many cell nuclei.

The muscle which is found in the walls of the blood vessels and intestines is "smooth"; that is, it has no striations. It is made up of spindle-shaped, mononuclear cells.

---

[1]) Connective tissue fibres on the other hand do not live. They are deposited in the inter-cellular matrix by the sparse connective tissue parent cells. It is the fibres, not the cells, that determine the mechanical properties of connective tissue. So called collagenous fibres (or fibrils) have great tensile strength and impart this properly to tendons and liga-ments and to such structures in the heart as the valves, the chordae tendineae and the annulus fibrosus.

Elastic fibres have not the same tensile strength as has collagen. They can sustain an increase in length to as much as three times the original measurement. They consti-tute the main part of the walls of the great arteries like the aorta which can thus change their volume so as to accommodate varying amounts of blood. Whereas the essential feature of connective tissue is the intercellular substance and its fibres, in muscular tissue it is the cellular components which give the tissue its character. The fine collagen fibrils which connect these cells, the endomysium, form only a very small part of the total volume.

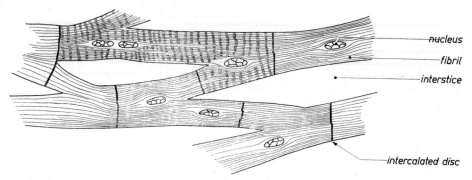

Fig. 66. Muscle cells of the heart, forming a network (diagrammatic; the cross-striations are shown in one segment only).

The striated fibre is enclosed in a sheath, the *sarcolemma*, consisting of a layer of fine collagenous fibrils embedded in interfibrillar substance and the cell membrane proper. The muscle fibre cytoplasm which it encloses is called *sarcoplasm*. In the sarcoplasm run the *myofibrils*, parallel with the long axis of the fibre. These myofibrils are the true contractile elements.

The myofibrils of striated muscle are regularly segmented, the segments differing in optical properties, staining properties, etc. The light bands which are only slightly birefringent are called isotropic or *I* bands; the dark portions, strongly birefringent, are called anisotropic or *A* bands. The *I* bands of one fibril lie next to the *I* bands of adjacent fibrils so that the whole muscle fibre appears to be striped. This striped effect is added to by the *Z* disc (Krause's membrane) which is seen as a thin dark line cutting across the isotropic bands and appears to be connected to the sarcolemma. The *Z* discs separate the fibril into a series of *sarcomeres*; each sarcomere thus consists of a *Z* disc, half an *I* band, an *A* band, half an *I* band and a *Z* disc (Fig. 67).

The individual myofibrils can be seen under the microscope. By electron microscopy it can be seen that each mybrofibril is a bundle of much finer fibrils called *myofilaments*. There are two types of filaments: thick ones restricted to the *A* bands and thin ones which run along the *I* band through the *Z* disc and eventually pass between the thick filaments in the *A* band for part of the distance. In contraction these thin filaments are apparently thrust between the thick filaments of the *A* band.

The impulse for contraction of the myofibrils is provided by the transmitted depolarisation of the cell membrane. This electrical phenomenon is basic to the study of electrocardiography. Electron microscopy has shown that there

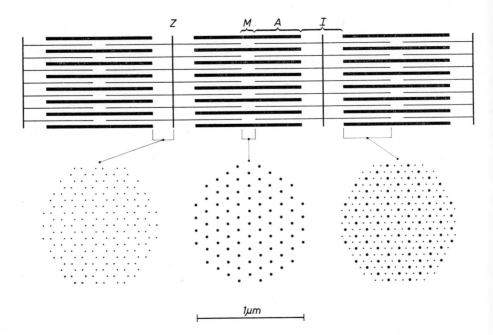

Fig. 67. Cross-striations and filaments (electron-microscopical view, diagrammatic)
Upper part: longitudinal section
Lower part: cross-section through the I, the M and the A band respectively.

are invaginations in the cell membrane at the point of attachment of the
Z discs and that the Z discs constitute a system of tubules which extend deep
into the sarcoplasm between the myofibrils. The hypothesis has been put
forward that the membrane of these tubes running in the interior of the fibre
plays the same role as that of the cell membrane on the exterior of the fibre,
i.e. transmission of the stimulus. This would explain how the peripheral and
central myofibrils of one fibre can respond almost synchronously to a
stimulus.

The fibres of the atrio-ventricular bundle and the sinu-atrial and atrio-
ventricular nodes are different from ordinary cardiac muscle fibres in that
the transverse striation is indistinct and that the myofibrils are peripherally
situated. The transmission of impulses along these fibres takes place approximately ten times as rapidly as along other myocardial fibres. The myocardium and the conducting system have a nerve supply but it is not thought
that normal transmission of impulses governing the spread of contraction
from one part of the heart to another takes place along neural fibres.

15.3 Electrophysiology

According to the previous description each of the heart muscle fibres can be considered as a small cylinder about 50 μm in cross-section, with a semi-permeable membrane 70 to 80 Å thick for a wall, which membrane has very special properties. An old concept that still has sense describes the fibre as a cylindrical capacitor with the membrane as insulator. In the polarised state it is negative on the inside and positively charged on the outside (Fig. 68), thus giving rise to a specific membrane voltage. Under certain conditions a "breakdown" occurs at some site so that the membrane becomes conductive.

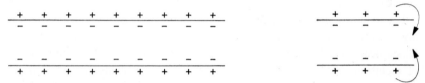

Fig. 68. Muscle fibre in polarised condition ("charged capacitor")

Fig. 69. At a breakdown point the "capacitor" discharges

The capacitor then discharges there (Fig. 69) so that the potential difference is leveled. The membrane now has the special property that it becomes conductive — "breaks down" — when the voltage difference between the inner and outer surfaces of the fibre drops below a certain value. (This is in contrast to the behaviour of an ordinary capacitor which breaks down when the voltage rises above a limiting value.) This phenomenon accounts for the process that with the start of an excitation anywhere at a point, the disturbance of equilibrium is propagated as a wave along the whole fibre thus producing electrical activity.

We shall discuss some details of this roughly sketched outline and in doing so must penetrate the innermost part of our object. The most common experimental method will be examined as above before reporting the experimental results.

To penetrate a muscle fibre an extremely thin needle electrode is required. This has been devised as a drawn glass tube whose diameter at the tip is reduced to 1 μm, open at both ends and filled with an electrolyte, for example potassium chloride. To prevent insurmountable resistance the tube is widened immediately beyond the tip (Fig. 70). Notwithstanding, the total resistance of such an electrode is of the order of 10 MΩ so that high input impedance requirements of the measuring apparatus must be established.

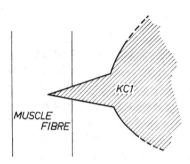

Fig. 70. Glass electrode inserted in a muscle fibre

Fortunately the voltages to be measured are not too small, being round about 0.1 volt.

Let us consider first the resting state, that is the situation in which the myocardium is polarised. How then does the capacitor become charged? It has been found that the K^+ ion plays an important part in the build up of membrane potential. It has been established by measurement that the K^+ concentration inside the fibre is many times higher than that outside. If we proceed in theory from an electrically neutral state (i.e. the same potential on either side of the membrane) then, because the K^+ ions pass through the fibre wall and the other ions cannot, a diffusion of K^+ ions to the outside occurs because the potassium concentration there is minimal. Consequently there is a surplus of anions remaining in the fibre, which causes the development of an electric field which will draw potassium ions back until the diffusion is exactly compensated i.e. until a steady state is reached. If we select an x-coordinate perpendicular to the membrane which is positive on the inside, we can describe the potassium transport to the outside, applying the law of diffusion:

$$m_K = -D \frac{dC}{dx} \qquad (15.1)$$

in which m_K is the quantity of K^+ ions transported per unit of time and per unit of surface, D is the diffusion constant and dC/dx is the concentration gradient across the membrane.

From physical chemistry it follows that the absolute value of potassium transport in the opposite direction is

$$m_K = \beta e C \frac{dV}{dx} \qquad (15.2)$$

where β is the mobility of the ions and e is the elementary charge. In the stationary state of course

$$-D \frac{dC}{dx} = \beta eC \frac{dV}{dx}. \tag{15.3}$$

By integration of this differential equation it follows that for the difference of potential between the inside and the outside of the membrane

$$\triangle V = \frac{D}{\beta e} \ln \frac{C_1}{C_2} \tag{15.4}$$

where C_1 is the potassium concentration inside and C_2 the concentration outside the membrane.

We see from (15.4) that the membrane potential is proportional to the log of the ratio of concentrations. If we examine this ratio in various species of animals, it appears that the variations are such that no difference of membrane potential greater than a factor of 3 is to be anticipated. This has indeed been verified.

We now consider what happens in excitation. As already observed, as a result of excitation the membrane (the fibre wall) suddenly becomes conductive and a breakdown takes place in it which is propagated from its point of origin along the whole fibre. Is is an obvious assumption that at the time of the discharge the voltage of the "capacitor" is zero. However this appears to be incorrect: the voltage changes sign and reaches about ¼ of its initial value (hence the interior becomes positive, the outside negative) as seen in Fig. 71 where the voltage over the membrane at a specific location is represented as a function of time. The dotted line in the figure is the zero line. The form of the potential curve is specific for the type of fibre, i.e., for myocardium, Purkinje system and atrioventricular node there are different curves. We shall not consider the entire course of the curve in detail but limit ourselves to the sudden potential jump at its inception.

How will the electric field appear as the result of excitation? The dipole layer is broken open as a result of the breakdown. Let us now examine a

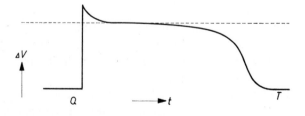

Fig. 71. The potential curve as can be measured in a certain point of a muscle fibre

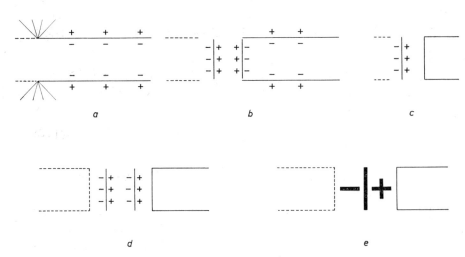

Fig. 72. The distribution of charge in a muscle fibre gives rise to a dipole, the origin of the heart vector

fibre on that side of the breakdown where rest conditions still prevail (Fig. 72*a*). We can then think of the opening as filled with two double layers, with oppositely directed charge (Fig. 72*b*). The right hand layer fills the gap in the membrane, so that a closed dipole layer is formed. As mentioned earlier (page 00) the field at the outside of such a closed dipole layer must be zero. The second layer, only provided to keep the total charge unaltered, then presents a fictitious dipole layer (Fig. 72*c*). A similar reasoning applied to the excited part of the fibre (with reversed charge distribution) also yields one resultant dipole layer (Fig. 72*d*). We now let these two like directed dipole layers fuse so that we have one single dipole layer over the whole fibre cross-section (Fig. 72*e*).

We may recall that the myocardium consists of a network of muscle fibres. In this network a well defined "fibre architecture" can be discerned, there are preferential directions so that in a particular region the fibres run mainly parallel to each other.

Since the fibres are almost simultaneously stimulated by the Purkinje system, we can conceive how the excitation front, hence the dipole layer, comes into existence and move through the heart during the duration of the heart beat.

For the sake of simplicity we did not consider in the above the part played by the sodium ion, also certain phenomena are left partially unexplained. We felt that a treatment of them lay beyond the scope of the present paper.

CHAPTER 16

CLINICAL APPLICATION
OF VECTORCARDIOGRAPHY

16.1 Genesis of the vectorcardiogram

From what was said in the previous chapter, it is clear that the distribution of the stimulus throughout the heart muscle by the conduction system and the arrangement of the muscle fibres in the syncytial network determine the conformation and direction of the dipole front and its progress through the heart muscle.

The first depolarisation occurs in the septum, taking its origin from fibres of the left bundle branch and spreading from left to right. Since the Purkinje fibres run along the endocardial surface of the ventricular wall, the endocardial side is excited first. The epicardial surface is reached as the result of muscle conduction. The first break-through (after about 25 ms) to the epicardium occurs where the septum abuts on the anterior wall near the apex. Subsequent spread is centrifugal from the apex. In this way the moving dipole front varies in time and place, determining in turn the "heart vector".

The manner of spread via the specialised conducting system has a strong determining effect on the behaviour of the vector. But peripheral conduction through the muscle itself is of considerable significance also. When the thickness of the muscle is locally increased the spread takes longer and this affects the direction of the vector; there may also be an increase in size of the vector, provided that the fibres of the wall be excited simultaneously. On the other hand the situation arises, when the depolarisation fronts in two groups of fibres move in opposite directions, that the resultant forces cancel each other out. When the muscle masses concerned are not equal an external effect will remain.

If the myocardium were a sphere with uniform wall thickness throughout, within which sphere a concentric front moved, nothing would be perceptible. In effect it more closely resembles a hemisphere because the atria are excited earlier and the mass of the atria is negligible compared with the ventricles. Furthermore, the walls are not of equal thickness: the left ventricle being approximately 3 times as thick as the right ventricle. For this reason a central symmetrical or an axially symmetrical spread of the front is excluded. As a rough approximation a plane of symmetry may be assumed that bisects the right and left ventricles. It has been thought that the potentials on either side of this plane of symmetry practically cancel each other out, so that the heart vector moves principally in the plane of symmetry, thus explaining the fact that the spatial vector loop is more or less planar. This would require, however, that the conduction system conforms to this plane of symmetry, which again is only approximately true.

If one studies the course of the action potential in Fig. 71, one sees that depolarisation, represented by the upstroke of the tracing, is a fast phenomenon (about 200 V per second). Contrarily, repolarisation, represented mainly by the rapid part of the downstroke, is slow. The speed of repolarisation (slope of downstroke) and the length of time during which the fibre is depolarised (width of the action potential) may vary from area to area in the heart, and may be dependent on the prevailing local metabolic conditions. It is unlikely that there is propagation of the repolarisation stimulus. Thus, the local characteristics of the action potential will affect the course of repolarisation throughout the heart, and due to these factors the repolarisation wave does not behave as one would expect. Its spread does not mimick the spread of activation, but rather the reverse, as is brought out by the agreement between the directions of the main repolarisation and main depolarisation vectors (less than 90° deviation, instead of the 180° difference one would anticipate).

The complexity of the anatomical and physiological framework in which the electrical processes occur is such that the form of the VCG could hardly be predicted. One had to proceed empirically. The same applies, and much stronger so, for the pathological VCG. Only recently have attempts been successful, in selected cases, to reconstruct the vectorcardiogram from data on the spread of excitation obtained with intramural needle electrodes.

16.2 Analysis of the normal vectorcardiogram

We will briefly analyse the VCG as it appears in the three orthogonal projections (frontal, horizontal and left-sagittal) (Fig. 73).

The ventricular depolarisation- or QRS-complex is preceded by the P wave (atrial contraction) and followed by the T wave (repolarisation of the ventricles). The three loops overlap at their origin so that for a detailed analysis of this part of the VCG it is necessary to magnify this portion or to break off the loop at a suitable point. In the frontal projection, the QRS vector loop runs "clockwise", in the horizontal and in the left-sagittal plane "anticlockwise". This is clearly an important phenomenon typical of the VCG, which is not manifest in the ECG, because in the ECG the temporal

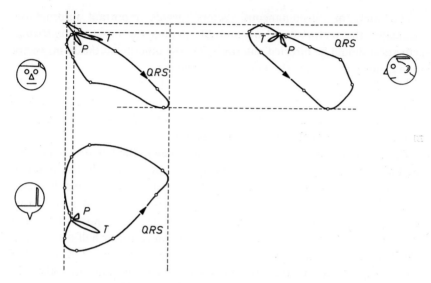

Fig. 73. Normal VCG in three projections
Time is marked by small circles every 10 ms.

relationship between the leads is neglected. As a general rule, a normal *QRS* loop lies approximately in one plane. (One might think this plane coincides with the plane of symmetry — if any — of the heart, but in practice this is not so.) The sense of inscription of the loop in the projections is dependent on the position of the plane of the loop in space, and this latter is expressed by the polar vector. "Polar vector" and "sense of inscription" are two different ways of describing the same phenomenon.

Furthermore, the "axis" of the loop is important. This is a rather loosely used term in diagnostic evaluation, meaning the preferred direction of the loop. It can be more sharply defined by making use of the direction of the gradient (whose determination from the VCG, unless done electronically, requires time-consuming measurement and calculation, however) of the "half-area vector", of the maximum spatial vector and still other expedients. One should realize that these magnitudes when determined in the projections are not necessarily identical with their spatial counterparts.

The relationship between the portions to the left and to the right of the origin (normally about 90 : 10) may also be important, as is the relationship between portions that are ahead and behind and above and below.

Attention must also be given to special shapes, irregularities, "bites", folds, delays etc. and to the moment of their occurrence.

The study of "instantaneous vectors" yields important information. Normally, the vectors at 10 ms and 20 ms after the onset of ventricular activation should be directed anteriorly. On the other hand the 30 ms vector should not point above the horizontal plane etc.

The QRS complex lasts about 100 ms. The distribution of time over the loop in this interval is to be read in the crowding of the time marks. Normally the largest speed of inscription is between the 40 and 60 ms time marks. There is a slight terminal retardation.

The T loop normally is inscribed anticlockwise in the horizontal and left-sagittal projections, clockwise in the frontal projection. It has a rather regular, elongated shape and due to this, maximum vector and half-area vector generally coincide. The outgoing limb is inscribed at a somewhat lesser speed than the returning limb, which will produce some difference in direction between the gradient and the maximum vector or half-area vector. The "axis", in whichever way identified, deviates somewhat from the QRS axis and is directed to the left and slightly anteriorly and inferiorly. The transition point where the QRS loop joins the T loop is called the Junction or J point. In normal cases the J point practically coincides with the point of origin, or E point, of the vectorcardiogram, in other words the T loop is closed, as well as the QRS loop.

It is useful to supplement the VCG with the recording of the simultaneous X, Y and Z components of the vector. These time-functions are something very close to electrocardiograms. The X component may be compared to leads I or V_6, the Z component to lead V_2, the Y component to lead aVF. However, they are certainly not identical with these leads! The classic ECG cannot be derived as such from the VCG, although it is very instructive to keep the VCG in mind for a better understanding of the ECG pattern. The components, on the other hand are nothing else but the VCG 'n another representation; they are truly orthogonal, lack proximity (i.e. multipole) effects, in short have all the features proper to the VCG.

16.3 The pathological VCG

Pathological variations are caused by:
1. Alteration of the *mass distribution* of heart muscle, in other words by a too much or a too little of muscle tissue;
2. Alteration of the *time schedule* of the activation of the heart muscle, due to change of the moment of initiation or of the duration of the depolarisation;

3. Alteration of the *electrical conductivity* of the surroundings of the heart, or by combinations of these factors.

16.3.1 ALTERATION OF THE MASS DISTRIBUTION

16.3.1.1. A "too little" of muscle tissue may be caused by an infarction. This means the obstruction of a branch of a coronary artery with subsequent death of the muscle area supplied by this branch.

An infarction manifests itself in the VCG by the absence of a deviation that is expected to occur at that moment of the cycle in a normal heart (Fig. 74*a* and 74*b*). In anteroseptal infarction, for example, in the first 20 ms of the *QRS*-complex the anteriorly directed vectors that are normally present

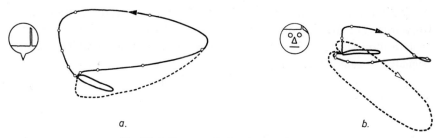

a.   *b.*

Fig. 74. Influence of infarction on the VCG
(dashed line: normal curve)
a: anterior-wall infarction
b: inferior-wall infarction

have disappeared. This must be due to the fact that the early activated antero-septal region, now being the seat of an infarction, does not make a contri-bution any more to the heart vector. In inferior wall infarction the initial vectors remain superiorly directed for a time longer than the usual maximum period of 30 ms, which presumably derives from the failure of inferiorly located tissue to take part in the activation process. Infarction causes other disturbances as well: conduction abnormalities related to "alterations of the time schedule" of the activation, in turn caused by detours in the pathways of depolarisation imposed by the infarction, and repolarisation anomalies mainly caused by the changes in properties of diseased muscle fibres. (*J* point displacement and *T* axis deviation.)

16.3.1.2. A "too much" of muscle is designated as "hypertrophy" and occurs when there is a pressure or a volume overload of a chamber of the heart.

Left Ventricular Hypertrophy (LVH) may result from narrowing of the aortic valve (aortic stenosis). In order to maintain a blood pressure that is adequate to supply blood to the tissues at an acceptable level, the left ventricle must produce a systolic pressure higher than normal, for example 240 mm Hg instead of 120 mm Hg. There is thus a pressure overload. When on the contrary the aortic valve leaks in the absence of stenosis (pure aortic insufficiency) a quantity of blood regurgitates from the aorta back to the left ventricle in diastole. This extra volume of blood must be pumped out at each heart beat without contributing to the circulating volume. This is volume overload which also leads to hypertrophy.

The VCG in LVH is characterised by the dominance after about 20 ms of those vectors that are directed to the left, posteriorly and somewhat superiorly. This leads to an increase of the left/right ratio, turning of the *QRS* "axis" towards the back, anticlockwise inscription of the frontal projection and coupled with it shifting of the polar vector upwards and forwards. The loop becomes somewhat pear shaped. In serious cases, repolarisation changes (*J* point shift, *T* axis deviation) occur which are designated "strain" (Fig. 75).

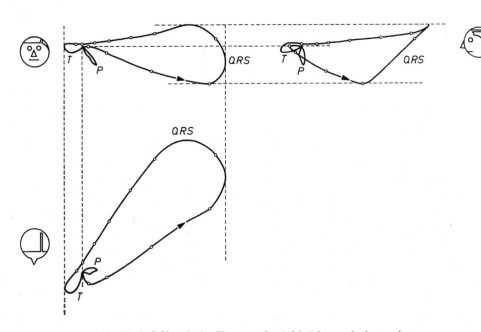

Fig. 75. Left Ventricular Hypertrophy (with left-ventricular strain).

The same is true of Right Ventricular Hypertrophy (RVH). Here pulmonary stenosis or insufficiency may be the cause. The VCG of RVH is characterised by predominance of those vectors after about 30 ms which are to the right, anterior and inferior. This leads to a decrease of the left/right ratio, turning of the QRS "axis" towards the right and anteriorly, clockwise inscription of the horizontal projection and coupled with it a shifting of the polar vector backwards and downwards. The loop becomes somewhat slipper shaped. In severe cases there are also T and J point deviations, having opposite direction to those of left ventricular strain, and labelled right ventricular strain (Fig. 76).

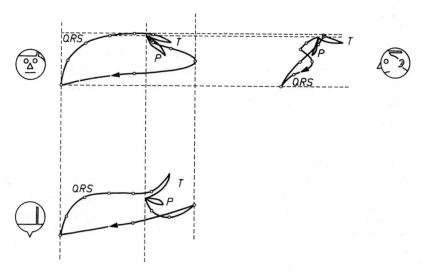

Fig. 76. Right Ventricular Hypertrophy (with right-ventricular strain)

LVH can be caused by mitral insufficiency and by septal defects as well as aortic valve disease. In such cases the left ventricular efficiency of work is diminished (blood regurgitates into the left auricle or right ventricle) so that volume overload has to occur to keep the circulating blood volume normal.

Mitral insufficiency through congestion in the pulmonary circulation can also lead to RVH; mitral stenosis has the same effect.

Ventricular septal defects, in addition to LVH cause RVH via volume and pressure overload (the left ventricle ejects blood into the right ventricle raising its pressure to, for example, 120 mm Hg as compared with the normal of about 35 mm Hg systolic).

An atrial septal defect on the contrary causes RVH exclusively by virtue of volume overload, because blood flows from the left atrium via the right atrium into the right ventricle which is passively distended more readily than the left ventricle because of its thinner wall. The extra circulating blood volume does not reach the left ventricle and hence causes no overload there.

Hypertrophy of the auricular wall is also possible (in mitral stenosis or insufficiency, tricuspid stenosis or insufficiency and atrial septal defect) but haemodynamically it is of less importance.

16.3.2 ALTERATION OF THE TIME SCHEDULE

In the case of "too much" muscle tissue, in addition to the increased mass, the increased duration of the excitation phase in the hypertrophied region also plays a role. By simply disturbing the time schedule of excitation the whole appearance of the VCG may change. When this factor is the only one altered we speak of disturbance of conduction.

16.3.2.1. When for example the atrioventricular node or the bundle of His do not transmit the stimulus arriving from the atrium, the condition is designated complete atrioventricular block. In cases like this the ventricles have to contract autonomously, independently of the Sinu-auricular pacemaker (otherwise the patient would die); this is initiated by the establishment of a secondary pacemaker somewhere in one of the ventricles. It is obvious that under these conditions the activation pattern will be overthrown completely and the appearance of the VCG will be affected in a way that is unpredictable.

16.3.2.2. If the interruption is situated in the right bundle branch (Right Bundle Branch Block, RBBB) then the septum and the left ventricle will be excited normally but the right ventricle will not be excited by the specific stimulus conducted through the specialized conducting tissue but rather by the slower muscle conduction. When the left ventricle is excited as a whole, the right ventricle is still depolarising in an intricate and delayed fashion. The VCG expresses this in a *QRS* loop of longer duration (greater than 120 ms for complete RBBB) with a characteristic trunklike, sluggishly traced deformation to the right and anteriorly (Fig. 77a).

By disturbance of the temporal sequence of depolarisation, repolarisation is similarly disturbed, with a resultant change of the *T* loop.

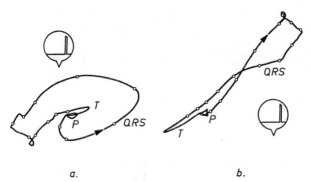

Fig. 77 *a*. Right bundle branch block
b. Left bundle branch block

16.3.2.3. Left Bundle Branch Block (LBBB) leads by analogy to increased duration (greater than 120 ms in complete LBBB) and a change in axis to the left, backwards and upwards. Vectors to the right are almost absent because septal excitation occurs from the right bundle branch in a leftward direction. Secondary *T* loop changes also occur (Fig. 77*b*).

16.3.3 ALTERATION OF ELECTRICAL CONDUCTIVITY

Changes in tissues in the vicinity of the heart in general have the effect of increasing electrical resistance, for example in chronic constrictive pericarditis (an additional layer of connective tissue surrounds the heart) and in emphysema (overdistended and aerated lungs). The result is "low voltage" in the ECG leads and a small VCG loop.

16.3.4. As a noteworthy example of the application of the VCG clinically we might consider atrial septal defect. There are two varieties, the socalled "secundum" (or dorsal) defect and the "primum" (or ventral) defect. The first is uncomplicated, while the second is in the region of the atrioventricular valves and accompanied by deformity of this valves and sometimes by ventricular septal defect. The difference in behaviour results from a differing embryological genesis. The primum defect is more malignant, more difficult to repair and requires the use of a heart-lung machine during surgery. It is thus of great importance that the differential diagnosis can be accurately established. Here the VCG, quite unexpectedly, plays an important part (Fig. 78*a* and 78*b*).

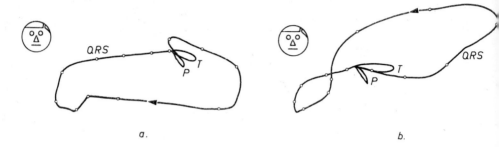

Fig. 78. Difference between auricular septal defects
a: Secundum defect
b: Primum defect. In both cases a Right Bundle Branch Block is also present.

The loops in the two conditions are completely different. In the one condition the frontal projection moves clockwise and in the other anticlockwise. The polar vector in the secundum defect is behind the meridian of 0-180° while in the primum defect it is in front. The characteristic appearance of the loops is independent of the presence of hypertrophy and appears to be caused by an anomalous "Anlage" of the conducting system at the time of embryonic development, in connection with the developmental anomaly of the septum.

In the ECG this diagnosis can be made with much less ease because calculating the time relationship between the leads is a troublesome and unreliable operation. It is the intrinsic property of the VCG that it represents this phase relationship in an unambiguous way.

BIBLIOGRAPHY
Prof. Dr. H. C. Burger

H. C. BURGER
On the Evaporation from a Circular Surface of a Liquid, Proc. Acad. Amsterd. **21** (1917) 271.

Over de verdamping van een cirkelvormig vloeistofoppervlak, Versl. Akad. Amsterd. **26** (1917) 1057.

On the Theory of the Brownian Movement and the Experiments of Brillouin, Proc. Acad. Amsterd. **20** (1918) 642.

Over de theorie der Brown'sche beweging en de proeven van Brillouin, Versl. Akad. Amsterd. **26** (1918) 1482.

(L. S. ORNSTEIN en H. C. BURGER)
Over de theorie der Brown'sche beweging, Versl. Akad. Amsterd. **27** (1918) 407.

Oplossen en groeien van kristallen, Thesis Utrecht, 1918.

Das Leitvermögen verdünnter mischkristallfreier Legierungen, Physik. Zs. **20** (1919) 73.

De grensconditie bij oplossen en kristalliseren, Hand. Ned. Nat. Gen. Congres, 1919, p. 81.

(L. S. ORNSTEIN and H. C. BURGER)
On the Theory of the Brownian Motion, Proc. Acad. Amsterd. **21** (1919) 922.

(L. S. ORNSTEIN en H. C. BURGER)
Statistiek van getallenreeksen, Versl. Akad. Amsterd. **27** (1919) 1146.

(L. S. ORNSTEIN en H. C. BURGER)
Frequentiewetten voor continu veranderlijke grootheden, Versl. Akad. Amsterd. **28** (1919) 183.

The Process of Solidification as a Problem of Conduction of Heat, Proc. Acad. Amsterd. **23** (1920) 616.

Observations of the Temperature during Solidification, Proc. Acad. Amsterd. **23** (1920) 691.

(and P. H. VAN CITTERT)
Measurements on the Intensity of Spectrum Lines by the Aid of the Echelon, Proc. Acad. Amsterd. **23** (1920) 790.

(L. S. ORNSTEIN en H. C. BURGER)
Photochemische reactie en straling, Versl. Akad. Amsterd. **29** (1920) 37.

Het stollingsproces als een probleem van warmtegeleiding, Versl. Akad. Amsterd. **29** (1920) 276.

Temperatuurwaarnemingen bij stolling, Versl. Akad. Amsterd. **29** (1920) 288.

(en P. H. VAN CITTERT)
Intensiteitsmetingen van spectraallijnen met behulp van het echelon, Versl. Akad. Amsterd. **29** (1920) 394.

(L. S. ORNSTEIN en H. C. BURGER)
De absorbtie-coëfficiënt van Jodium-oplossingen in het zichtbare spectrum, I, Versl. Akad. Amsterd. **29** (1920) 573.

(P. H. VAN CITTERT und H. C. BURGER)
Einfluß der Temperatur auf Stellung und Intensität der Stufengitterlinien, Physik. Zs. **21** (1920) 16.

De structuur van getrokken wolfraamdraden, Physica, Ned. T. Natuurk. **1** (1921) 214.

Das Leitvermögen verdünnter mischkristallfreier Legierungen (Zur Erwiderung an Herrn K. Lichtenecker), Physik. Zs. **22** (1921) 28.

Struktur des Wolframs, Physik. Zs. **23** (1922) 14.

Glijvlakken in tinkristallen, Physica, Ned. T. Natuurk. **2** (1922) 26.

Bepaling van de dichtheid van wolfraam met behulp van röntgenstralen, Physica, Ned. T. Natuurk. **2** (1922) 114.

(L. S. ORNSTEIN en H. C. BURGER)
Ionisatie in sterrenatmosferen, Physica, Ned. T. Natuurk. **2** (1922) 308.

(L. S. ORNSTEIN und H. C. BURGER)
Zur Theorie des Schroteffektes, Ann. d. Phys. **70** (1923) 622.

(L. S. ORNSTEIN und H. C. BURGER)
Die Dimension der Einsteinschen Lichtquanten, Zs. f. Phys. **20** (1923) 345.

(L. S. ORNSTEIN und H. C. BURGER)
Zur Dynamik des Stoßes zwsichen einem Lichtquant und einem Elektron, Zs. f. Phys. **20** (1923) 351.

Het onderwijs in de natuurkunde aan de studenten in de geneeskunde, Openbare les gehouden te Utrecht op 11 oktober 1922. (Verkort), Physica, Ned. T. Natuurk. **3** (1923) 1.

Berekening van kristalstructuren uit röntgenogrammen Physica, Ned. T. Natuurk. **3** (1923) 121.

(L. S. ORNSTEIN und H. C. BURGER)
Zusammenwirken von Lichtquanten und Plancksches Gesetz, Zs. f. Phys. **21** (1924) 358.

(und H. B. DORGELO)
Beziehung zwischen inneren Quantenzahlen und Intensitäten von Mehrfachlinien, Zs. f. Phys. **23** (1924) 258.

(L. S. ORNSTEIN und H. C. BURGER)
Strahlungsgesetz und Intensität von Mehrfachlinien, Zs. f. Phys. **24** (1924) 41.

(L. S. ORNSTEIN und H. C. BURGER)
Die Feinstruktur der gelben Heliumlinie 5876 Å, Zs. f. Phys. **26** (1924) 57.

(L. S. ORNSTEIN und H. C. BURGER)
Intensitäten der Komponenten im Zeemaneffekt, Zs. f. Phys. **28** (1924) 135.

(L. S. ORNSTEIN und H. C. BURGER)
Nachschrift zu der Arbeit: Intensitäten der Komponenten im Zeemaneffekt, Zs. f. Phys. **29** (1924) 241.

(L. S. ORNSTEIN und H. C. BURGER)
Lichtbrechung und Zerstreuung nach der Lichtquantentheorie, Zs. f. Phys. **30** (1924) 253.

(L. S. ORNSTEIN und H. C. BURGER)
Die Polarisation des Resonanzlichts, Physik. Zs. **25** (1924) 298.

(en L. S. ORNSTEIN)
Stralingsformule en lichtquanta, Physica, Ned. T. Natuurk. **4** (1924) 52.

(W. J. H. MOLL, H. C. BURGER and J. VAN DER BILT)
The Distribution of the Energy over the Sun's Disc, Bull. Astr. Instit. Netherl. **3** (1925) 83.

(W. J. H. MOLL and H. C. BURGER)
A New Vacuum Thermo-Element, Phil. Mag. **50** - 6th series (1925) 618.

(W. J. H. MOLL and H. C. BURGER)
The Thermo-Relay, Phil. Mag. **50** - 6th series (1925) 624.

(W. J. H. MOLL and H. C. BURGER)
The Sensitivity of a Galvanometer and its Amplification, Phil. Mag. **50** - 6th series (1925) 626.

(L. S. ORNSTEIN und H. C. BURGER)
Intensität von Multiplettlinien, Zs. f. Phys. **31** (1925) 355.

(W. J. H. MOLL und H. C. BURGER)
Ein neues Vakuumthermoelement, Zs. f. Phys. **32** (1925) 575.

(L. S. ORNSTEIN und H. C. BURGER)
Dispersion nach der Lichtquantentheorie, Zs. f. Phys. **32** (1925) 678.

(L. S. ORNSTEIN, H. C. BURGER und W. C. VAN GEEL)
Intensitäten der Komponenten im Zeemaneffekt, Zs. f. Phys. **32** (1925) 681.

(W. J. H. MOLL und H. C. BURGER)
Das Thermorelais, Zs. f. Phys. **34** (1925) 109.

(W. J. H. MOLL und H. C. BURGER)
Empfindlichkeit und Leistungsfähigkeit eines Galvanometers, Zs. f. Phys. **34** (1925) 112.

(W. J. H. MOLL und H. C. BURGER)
Leerboek der Natuurkunde, I, P. Noordhof N.V., Groningen, 1926.

(W. J. H. MOLL und H. C. BURGER)
Leerboek der Natuurkunde, II, P. Noordhof N.V., Groningen, 1927.

(L. S. ORNSTEIN und H. C. BURGER)
Intensität verbotener Multipletts, Naturwiss. **15** (1927) 670.

(P. H. VAN CITTERT en H. C. BURGER)
Ware en schijnbare breedte van spectraallijnen, Physica, Ned. T. Natuurk. **7** (1927) 149.

(L. S. ORNSTEIN, H. C. BURGER, J. TAYLOR and W. CLARKSON)
The Brownian Movement of a Galvanometer Coil and the Influence of the Temperature of the Outer Circuit, Proc. R. Soc. A, **115** (1927) 391.

(L. S. ORNSTEIN und H. C. BURGER)
Die Einheit vom Singulett- und Triplettsystem und ihre Interkombinationen, Zs. f. Phys. **40** (1927) 403.

(und P. H. VAN CITTERT)
Wahre und scheinbare Breite von Spektrallinien, Zs. f. Phys. **44** (1927) 58.

(L. S. ORNSTEIN en H. C. BURGER)
Het ontstaan van het helium-spectrum, Physica, Ned. T. Natuurk. **8** (1928) 111.

(L. S. ORNSTEIN, H. C. BURGER und W. KAPUSCINSKI)
Das Entstehen des He-Spektrums bei elektrischer Anregung, Zs. f. Phys. **51** (1928) 34.

(und P. H. VAN CITTERT)
Verbreiterung von Spektrallinien durch Selbstabsorption, Zs. f. Phys. **51** (1928) 638.

(W. J. H. MOLL en H. C. BURGER)
Leerboek der Natuurkunde, III, P. Noordhof N.V., Groningen, 1928.

(L. S. ORNSTEIN und H. C. BURGER)
Intensitätsverhältnis von Balmer- und Paschenlinien, Zs. f. Phys. **62** (1930) 636.

(und P. H. VAN CITTERT)
Die Herstellung von Wismut-Antimon-Vakuumthermoelementen durch Verdampfung, Zs. f. Phys. **66** (1930) 210.

(en P. H. VAN CITTERT)
De vervaardiging van bismuth-antimoon vacuum-thermoëlementen door verdamping, Warmtetechniek **2** (1931) 1.

(L. S. ORNSTEIN und H. C. BURGER)
Eine Eichmethode für eine Normallampe mit Linienspektrum, Zs. f. Phys. **76** (1932) 777.

(und P. H. VAN CITTERT)
Wahre und scheinbare Intensitätsverteilung in Spektrallinien, Zs. f. Phys. **79** (1932) 722.

(L. S. ORNSTEIN, W. J. H. MOLL und H. C. BURGER)
Objektive Spektralphotometrie, Braunschweig, Vieweg, 1932.

(und P. H. VAN CITTERT)
Wahre und scheinbare Intensitätsverteilung in Spektrallinien, II, Zs. f. Phys. **81** (1933) 428.

(L. S. ORNSTEIN und H. C. BURGER)
Intensitätsverhältnis von Balmer- und Paschenlinien, II, Zs. f. Phys. **83** (1933) 177.

(und P. H. VAN CITTERT)
Bemerkung zu der Arbeit von L. Farkas und S. Levy: *Messung der Intensitätsverteilung und Breite von prädissoziierenden Linien des AlH-Moleküls*, Zs. f. Phys. **87** (1934) 545.

(und P. H. VAN CITTERT)
Bemerkung zu der Arbeit von L. Farkas und S. Levy: *Messung der Intensitätsverteilung und Breite von prädissoziierenden Linien des AlH-Moleküls, II*, Zs. f. Phys. **90** (1934) 70.

(und P. H. VAN CITTERT)
Die Einstellung der Koinzidenz beim Multiplexinterferenzspektroskop, Physica **2** (1935) 87.

(en P. H. VAN CITTERT)
Ware en schijnbare intensiteitsverdeling in spectraallijnen, Ned. T. Natuurk. **3** (1936) 170.

(J. B. VAN MILAAN and L. S. ORNSTEIN)
Intensity Measurements in the Spectrum of Helium, Physica **4** (1937) 730.

(and P. H. VAN CITTERT)
Intensity Measurements in Hyperfine Structure of the Mercury Line $6^3P_2 - 7^3S_1$ ($\lambda = 5461\ \mathring{A}U$) in Absorption, Physica **5** (1938) 177.

(G. C. E. BURGER and H. C. BURGER)
Determination of the Rate of Infection in Tuberculosis, Proc. Acad. Amsterd. **41** (1938) 611.

De grenzen van onze waarneming, Faraday **10** (1939) 122.

(en P. H. VAN CITTERT)
Hyperfijne structuur van spectraallijnen, Ned. T. Natuurk. **6** (1939) 169.

(and J. B. VAN MILAAN)
Measurement of the Reflective Power of Metallic Mirrors, Physica **6** (1939) 435.

(and P. H. VAN CITTERT)
Intensity Measurements of Helium Lines in Absorption, Physica **7** (1940) 13.

(W. J. H. MOLL und H. C. BURGER)
Thermoelektrische Vakuummeter, Zs. f. techn. Phys. **21** (1940) 199.

Het electrisch geleidingsvermogen van het menselijk lichaam, Natuur- en Gen. Congres, 1941.

(and J. B. VAN MILAAN)
Measurements of the Specific Resistance of the Human Body to Direct Current, Acta Med. Scand. **114** (1943) 584.

(en E. F. M. VAN DER HELD)
Warmte-afgifte van het menselijk lichaam in vochtige lucht, Ned. T. Geneesk. **87** (1943) 938.

(en P. H. VAN CITTERT)
Viscositeit van bloed tijdens stolling, Ned. T. Geneesk. **88** (1944) 760.

Medische Fysica, Standaarddictaat, 1946.

Fysische Meetmethodes, Dictaat, 1946.

(and J. B. VAN MILAAN)
Heart Vector and Leads, I, Brit. Heart J. **8** (1946) 157.

(G. C. E. BURGER en H. C. BURGER)
Het differentiële bloedbeeld en het toeval, Geneesk. Gids **26** (1946).

W. J. H. Moll (1876-1946), Ned. T. Natuurk. **12** (1946) 137.

Medische Fysica. Hoofdstuk 12 in: R. KRONIG (ed.), *Leerboek der Natuurkunde*, deel II, blz. 341. Scheltema & Holkema, Amsterdam, 1947.

(and J. B. VAN MILAAN)
Heart Vector and Leads, II, Brit. Heart J. **8** (1947) 154.

(A. CLARENBURG en H. C. BURGER)
Het koken van eendeneieren, Voeding **8** (1947) 126.

Physical Foundations of Vectorcardiography, Acta Med. Belgica **4** (1948) 61.

(and J. B. VAN MILAAN)
Heart Vector and Leads, III, Brit. Heart J. **10** (1948) 229.

(en G. C. E. BURGER)
Medische Fysica, N.V. Noordholl. Uitg. Mij., Amsterdam, 1949.

(and L. J. KOOPMAN)
On the Analysis and Origin of Heart Sounds, I, Acta Card. **4** (1949) 131.

(L. J. KOOPMAN and A. P. TH. OVEREEM)
On the Analysis and Origin of Heart Sounds, II, Acta Card. **5** (1950) 1.

(and F. L. J. JORDAN)
The Influence of Distance on the Pitch of the Percussion Note, Acta Med. Scand. **136** (1950) 283.

(and A. CLARENBURG)
The Killing of Salmonella Bacteria from Ducks' Eggs by Heating, Antonie v. Leeuwenhoek **16** (1950) 386.

(A. G. T. BECKING, H. C. BURGER and J. B. VAN MILAAN)
A Universal Vectorcardiograph, Brit. Heart J. **12** (1950) 339.

(A. CLARENBURG and H. C. BURGER)
Survival of Salmonellae in Boiled Ducks' Eggs, Food Res. **15** (1950) 340.

Gaswisseling tussen bloed en alveoli, Hand. Ned. Nat. Gen. Congres, 1951. p. 103.

(G. CASTELEYN and F. L. J. JORDAN)
How is Percussion done? Acta Med. Scand. **142** (1952) 108.

(R. BRAAMS and J. F. C. WERZ)
Depth-dose Data for Roentgen Radiation at 30-100 kilovolts, Acta Rad. **37** (1952) 531.

(J. B. VAN MILAAN and W. DEN BOER)
Comparison of Different Systems of Vectorcardiography, Brit. Heart J. **14** (1952) 401.

(en J. A. SMIT)
Schoolproeven: *8. Controle (ijking) van een wijzermanometer, 9. Dichtheidsmeting m.b.v. zwevende druppels*, Ned. T. Natuurk. **18** (1952) 314.

Grensgebied, Oratie gehouden op 12 mei 1952, Fys. Lab. m 2568.

(A. NOORDERGRAAF and A. M. W. VERHAGEN)
Physical Basis of the Low-Frequency Ballistocardiograph. I, Am. Heart J. **46** (1953) 71.

(en J. A. SMIT)
Schoolproeven, *17. Over een tiental proeven vnl. ontleend aan een eerstejaarspracticum te Utrecht*, Ned. T. Natuurk. **19** (1953) 348.

How much Physics? Proc. 1st World Conf. on Med. Educ. (London), 1953, p. 133.

(H. A. TOLHOEK and F. G. BACKBIER)
The Potential Distribution on the Body Surface caused by a Heart Vector, Am. Heart J. **48** (1954) 249.

The Zero of Potential: a Persistent Error, Am. Heart J. **49** (1955) 581.

(W. DEN BOER, H. C. BURGER and J. B. VAN MILAAN)
Vectorcardiograms of Normal and Premature Beats in Different Lead Systems, Brit. Heart J. **17** (1955) 1.

(Y. VAN DER FEER and J. H. DOUMA)
On the Theory of Cardiac Output Measurement by the Injection Method, Acta Card. **11** (1956) 1.

(J. B. VAN MILAAN and W. KLIP)
Comparison of two Systems of Vectorcardiography with an Electrode to the Frontal and Dorsal Sides of the Trunk, respectively, Am. Heart J. **51** (1956) 26.

(and A. NOORDERGRAAF)
Physical Basis of Ballistocardiography, II, Am. Heart J. **51** (1956) 127.

(and A. NOORDERGRAAF)
Physical Basis of Ballistocardiography. III, Am. Heart J. **51** (1956) 179.

(A. NOORDERGRAAF, J. J. M. KORSTEN and P. ULLERSMA)
Physical Basis of Ballistocardiography, IV, Am. Heart J. **52** (1956) 653.

(A. G. W. VAN BRUMMELEN and F. J. DANNENBURG)
Theory and Experiments on Schematized Models of Stenosis, Circ. Res. **4** (1956) 425.

De ontwikkeling van de medische fysica in Utrecht en elders, Ned. T. Natuurk. **22** (1956) 135.

A Theoretical Elucidation of the Notion "Ventricular Gradient", Am. Heart J. **53** (1957) 240.

(A. NOORDERGRAAF and H. J. L. KAMPS)
Physical Basis of Ballistocardiography, V, Am. Heart J. **53** (1957) 907.

Lead Vector Projections, I, Ann. New York Acad. Sc. **65** (1957) 1076.

(and J. P. VAANE)
A Criterion Characterizing the Orientation of a Vectorcardiogram in Space, Am. Heart J. **56** (1958) 29.

(J. B. VAN MILAAN and W. KLIP)
Comparison of Three Different Systems of Vectorcardiography, Am. Heart J. **57** (1959) 723.

(en J. A. SMIT)
P. H. van Cittert, 40 jaar doctor, Ned. T. Natuurk. **25** (1959) 1.

(H. W. HOREMAN and A. J. M. BRAKKEE)
Comparison of Some Methods for Measuring Peripheral Blood Flow, Phys. Med. Biol. **4** (1959) 168.

(and H. W. HOREMAN)
Physical Properties of Some Volume Recorders in Plethysmography, Phys. Med. Biol. **4** (1959) 176.

Opening speech, Proc. 1st Congr. Soc. for BCG Res., Zeist, 1960, p. 3.

A Physicist's View on the Ballistocardiographic Effect, Proc. 1st Congr. Soc. for BCG Res., Zeist, 1960, p. 32.

(A. G. W. VAN BRUMMELEN and G. VAN HERPEN)
Heart Vector and Leads, Am. Heart J. **61** (1961) 317.

Letter to the Editor, Am. Heart J. **61** (1961) 428.

(A. G. W. VAN BRUMMELEN and G. VAN HERPEN)
Compromise in Vectorcardiography, Displacement of Electrodes as a Means of Adapting One Lead System to Another, Am. Heart J. **62** (1961) 398.

(and R. VAN DONGEN)
Specific Electric Resistance of Body Tissues, Phys. Med. Biol. **5** (1961) 431.

The Strength of the Heart and the Energy Law, Proc. 2nd Eur. Symp. for Ballistocardiography, Bonn, 1961, p. 113.

(A. G. W. VAN BRUMMELEN and G. VAN HERPEN)
Compromise in Vectorcardiography, II. Alterations of Coefficients as a Means of Adapting One Lead System to Another, Am. Heart J. **64** (1962) 666.

Ballistocardiography and Vectorcardiography, Similarity and Difference, Proc. 3rd Eur. Symp. for Ballistocardiography, Brussels, 1962, p. 88.

Welcome and Introduction, In: Circulatory Analog Computers, p. 2, North-Holl. Publ. Comp., Amsterdam, 1963.

Models, In: Circulatory Analog Computers, p. 4, North-Holl. Publ. Comp., Amsterdam, 1963.

(A. NOORDERGRAAF und H. W. L. VONKEN)
Physikalische Betrachtungen über Elektroakupunktur, Hippokrates **34** (1963) 861.

Ballistocardiography and Vectorcardiography, Similarity and Difference, Transaction & Studies of the College of Physicians of Philadelphia. 4 Ser., Vol. 31, No. 4, April 1964 (Hatfield Lecture, Philadelphia, 6 november 1963).

(and A. G. W. VAN BRUMMELEN)
A Physicist's View on the Possibilities of Measurement of Stroke Volume by means of Physical Methods using Ultra Low Frequency BCG, IVe Congrès européen de balistocardiographie, Lille médicale 1964, numéro speciale p. 27-31.

(A. G. W. VAN BRUMMELEN and G. VAN HERPEN)
Correlation between Subjective and Objective Measures of Correspondence between Different Systems of Vectorcardiography, Am. Heart J. **67**, no. 4 (1964) 512.

Het begrip „arbeid" in natuurkunde, fysiologie en geneeskunde, Vijfde Einthoven-voordracht gehouden aan de Rijks-Universiteit te Leiden, 1964, 3-16.

Theses prepared with Prof. Dr. H. C. Burger

F. A. RODRIGO,
Experiments concerning the State of Chlorophyll in Plants, 4 july 1955.

A. NOORDERGRAAF,
Physical Basis of Ballistocardiography, 10 december 1956.

J. C. GOEDHEER,
Optical Properties and in Vivo Orientation of Photosynthetic Pigments, 11 february 1957.

G. VAN DEN BRINK
Retinal Summation and the Visibility of Moving Objects, 17 june 1957.

R. RIKMENSPOEL,
Photoelectric and Cinematographic Measurements of the "Motility" of Bull Sperm Cells, 11 november 1957.

B. F. VISSER,
Clinical Gas Analysis based on Thermal Conductivity, 9 december 1957.

H. W. HOREMAN,
Comparison of Methods for Measuring Peripheral Blood Flow, 27 january 1958.

Y. VAN DER FEER,
The Determination of Cardiac Output by the Injection Method, 24 february 1958.

J. N. VAN DER HORST
De normale reactie van de huidtemperatuur van de mens bij wisselende omgevingstemperaturen, 4 november 1958.

G. CASTELEYN,
Physical Investigations on Percussion, 20 november 1961.

A. G. W. VAN BRUMMELEN,
Some Applications of Digital Computing and Model Experiments of Haemodynamics, 13 december 1961.

DR. W. KLIP,
Velocity and Damping of "the Pulse Wave", 5 november 1962.

INDEX